The
Bristol Approach
to Living
with Cancer

The
Bristol Approach
to Living
with Cancer

New edition revised and updated by

HELEN COOKE

ROBINSON
London

Constable & Robinson Ltd
3 The Lanchesters
162 Fulham Palace Road
London W6 9ER
www.constablerobinson.com

First published in the UK by Robinson,
an imprint of Constable & Robinson Ltd, 2000

This new and revised edition published in the UK by
Robinson, an imprint of Constable & Robinson Ltd, 2003

A copy of the British Library Cataloguing in Publication Data
is available from the British Library.

ISBN 1–84119–680–0

Printed and bound in the EU

10 9 8 7 6 5 4 3 2 1

Dedication

This book is dedicated to Penny Brohn, and her supporter and co-founder of the Bristol Cancer Help Centre, Pat Pilkington.

Also to the thousands of people who have participated in the Bristol Approach since the Centre's doors opened – they continue to be great teachers and a real inspiration to us all.

Enormous appreciation must also go to all the staff at the Bristol Cancer Help Centre who have built on the founding principles and lovingly and dedicatedly continue to carry the work forward.

Contents

Foreword

Occasionally, Western medicine seems unsure of its own identity. The public is endlessly bombarded with propaganda heralding new, more powerful, more scientific, more hi-tech, more expensive treatment, today's latest scientific achievement or tomorrow's breakthrough. And why not? The improvements have been dazzling. The X-ray was developed only just over a century ago. Advances in medical technology followed an unceasing stream, including the electrocardiogram to monitor heart conditions and, from the 1920s, electron microscopes, permitting investigation of cell pathology. More recent years have brought endoscopes, lasers, ultrasound and scanners. And practical consequences have followed. One milestone was the first surgical intervention, just over 50 years ago, for 'blue babies' born with congenital heart disease. Open heart surgery dates from the 1950s; by-pass operations began in 1967. Surgery became like space travel, boldly going where none had gone before. Organ replacement was developed, first with kidneys, and heart transplants became banner headlines in 1967.

For the future, the Human Genome Project – the offspring of new theories and new scientific disciplines like molecular biology – affords us still further prospects of new breakthroughs. We already have a sound grasp of the genetic basis of terrible disorders like muscular dystrophy, Tay-Sachs disease, Huntington's disease, and cystic fibrosis. There is every likelihood that other crippling and fatal conditions will turn out to be genetically programmed, perhaps even some cancers. As in every other department of medicine, understanding is sure to lead to therapeutic action. Medicine has relieved humankind of many scourges; helped by the Genome Project, the twenty-first century seems set fair to be the age when the burden of genetic disorders is finally lifted.

But doctors, scientists and their publicists sometimes seem to forget that there is more to medicine than that. Medicine is an art as well as a science, and the healing art is holistic through and through. It must touch all aspects of the sick person – the mind as well as the body, the soul, spirit or feelings as well as the reason, and the unconscious as well as the conscious. And it must be interactive, a dialogue between the sick person and the healer. The word 'patient' comes from the Latin for passive, but it is vital that the patient should be an agent as well.

The holistic approach to health is widely associated with various sorts of 'alternative medicine', Western and Eastern alike. And rightly so. But they are also integral to the mainstream history of conventional medicine, and have been so ever since the Greeks immortally inscribed in the Hippocratic Oath the promise 'above all, to do no harm'.

The medicine of antiquity, which was transmitted to Islam and then back to the medieval West, and which remained powerful throughout the Renaissance, paid great attention to general health maintenance through regulation of diet, exercise, hygiene and lifestyle. In the absence of decisive anatomical and physiological expertise, and without the benefit of a powerful arsenal of cures and surgical skills, the ability to diagnose and make prognoses was highly valued, and an intimate physician–patient relationship was fostered. The teachings of antiquity – which remained authoritative into the eighteenth century and still supply reservoirs of medical folklore – were more successful in helping people to cope with chronic conditions, and in soothing lesser ailments, than in conquering the life-threatening infections that became endemic and epidemic in the civilized world – leprosy, plague, smallpox, measles, and, later, the 'filth diseases' (like typhus) associated with urban squalor.

This rather personal tradition of bedside medicine long remained popular in the West, as did its equivalents in Chinese and Ayurvedic medicine. But in Europe it was supplemented and challenged by the creation of a more 'scientific' type of medicine, grounded, for the first time, upon experimental anatomical and physiological investigation, epitomized, from the fifteenth century, by the dissection techniques that were to become central to medical education. Landmarks in this programme include the publication of *On the Fabric of the Human Body* (1543) by the Paduan professor, Andreas Vesalius, the first momentous anatomical atlas and a work that challenged truths received since Galen; and William Harvey's *On the Motion of the Heart* (1628), which put physiological enquiry on the map through experiments demonstrating the circulation of the blood and the role of the heart as a pump. Thereafter 'scientic medicine' took off.

But its achievements must not blind us to the fact that both sides of medicine – the humane and personal no less than the scientific – are equally important and central to our medical tradition. As this absorbing book shows, the Bristol Cancer Help Centre is dedicated to upholding and integrating both. In one light it may be viewed as pioneering 'alternative approaches', but these are, in their own way, central to what medicine has always been about.

Roy Porter
Wellcome Institute for the History of Medicine, London, 2000

Preface and Acknowledgements

The main reason for writing this book is to help people with cancer to understand the pivotal role they can play in their own healing and recovery process. In the minds of many people, cancer is a one-way street, and the diagnosis of cancer equates to a death sentence. This is very wrong. There are many people who recover from cancer and also documented cases of 'spontaneous remission' or 'remarkable recovery' from supposedly 'terminal' cancer. There is great variation, too, in the periods of remission or disease-free interval in people who apparently have the same sorts of cancer, and so it is clear that there are many factors other than medical treatments that determine whether one lives with, or dies from, cancer.

During the 20 years of work and study at the Bristol Cancer Help Centre, it has become clear that many of these factors are ones over which the individual can take control. Of these, probably the most important of all is taking control itself. Most obviously, this means becoming actively involved in your own care and management, i.e. taking yourself out of the passenger seat – the passive, dependent, patient role – and placing yourself firmly in the driving seat. The other factors are mediated through specific healthcare interventions, which all help to promote optimum health in the presence of illness, however severe the illness may be.

We hope that, in explaining how this active role can be assumed, this book will help people to find the hope, inspiration, support and guidance that will enable them to cope with the frightening challenge of their illness. More than this, it is hoped that through taking this approach, your experience of cancer may be transformed – as it has been for many – from a crisis into an opportunity, a chance to embark upon a far happier, healthier and more fulfilling lifestyle than you had before diagnosis.

The second aim is to address the vulnerability of those caring for people with cancer: to look at the stress and distress associated with their role, and legitimize their need for support and help. Supporters will be encouraged to protect themselves from the risks associated with the high demands and trauma of living with life-threatening illness in a loved one, to learn how to protect and care for themselves, and in so doing to maximize their ability to offer support and help to the one for whom they are caring.

In preparing this second edition I would like to acknowledge the therapy team of the Bristol Cancer Help Centre for the way they continue to lovingly support and inspire all those who attend courses. I would also like to record my enormous appreciation to those who made individual contributions (listed below). I would also like to acknowledge Dr Rosy Daniel, former Medical Director of the Centre, who wrote the first edition, and the late Professor Roy Porter, the foremost medical historian of our age, whose foreword to the first edition is reproduced here unchanged.

A very big thank you to Gillian Somerscales, who patiently and painstakingly copy-edited this edition. Enormous gratitude to Julia Kwan for her calm secretarial support and good humour throughout the process. Also to Chris Head, Pat Turton, Melissa Henry, Heather Martin and Lynda McGilvray for their support and input.

Helen Cooke MA, RGN, Dip Counselling
Director of Therapy, Bristol Cancer Help Centre, 2003

Members of the Therapy Team Who Made Contributions

Chapter 2: chapter written by Dr David Beales

Other contributors

Art Therapist	Diana Brueton
Counsellors	Ruth Benor, Maggie Peters
Doctor	Sara Miller
Healers	Janet Swan, Sue Alston
Bodyworkers	Andy Fagg, Janet MacDonald
Librarian	Chrissy Holmes
Music Therapist	Professor Leslie Bunt
Nurses	Eula Dunn, Katherine McKenzie
Nutritional Therapists	Ute Brookman, Cilla Moncrieff, Victoria Kubiak

PART ONE
Setting the Framework

1
The Bristol Approach

This chapter describes the approach of the Bristol Centre to the care of people with cancer, outlines the history of the Centre's foundation and development, and describes the programme of therapy and support it offers.

The Bristol Cancer Help Centre

The Bristol Cancer Help Centre's *raison d'être* is quite simply to offer healing and support both to people with any form of cancer and to those who support them. The Centre's approach (the Bristol Approach) is holistic in the sense that it recognizes the unity and interdependence of body, mind and spirit within each individual. The Centre seeks, first through the teaching of the holistic approach to health, and then by implementation of the holistic medical model, to help individuals achieve the optimum level of health for the remainder of their lives, however long or short a time that may be.

The first question many people who come to the Centre ask is, 'Can I use the Bristol Approach alongside orthodox medicine?' The answer is a resounding 'Yes'. In fact, integration of holistic and orthodox approaches is very likely to result in better treatment outcomes, reduced symptoms and side-effects of treatments, and overall a far greater sense of control and much improved quality of life than either route followed exclusively. The majority of people who come to the Centre opt for this 'best of both worlds' approach, although on rare occasions some choose an alternative approach only.

It is part of the Bristol Approach to support each individual in the choices and decisions he or she makes, and no pressure is placed on anybody to pursue any particular form or style of treatment, orthodox or complementary. Rather, the approach is to offer in-depth medical counselling, once the person has recovered from the shock of diagnosis, in order to make sure that the choices they are making are right for them. In fact, once time and unconditional support are given, and their fears are addressed, people may change their initial ideas about refusing treatment and accept conventional intervention.

The primary focus of the work at the Centre is the therapy services, but in addition to these the Centre has developed extensive educational and informational services, and these are available to people with cancer, their supporters, healthcare professionals and the general public.

Penny Brohn – co-founder of the Bristol Cancer Help Centre – lived with breast cancer for 20 years. In the pages that follow, you will read about many others who have made remarkable transformations to their lives. You will learn about the Bristol Approach to health and illness, the science underpinning it, and the different therapies and self-help techniques that you can use to strengthen your health, increase your tolerance of conventional treatments and enhance your chances of recovery whether or not you come to the Centre. It is hoped that this book will help you to recognize the crucial role that you can play in your recovery process, and, most important of all, that your sense of hope and control will begin to return. Many thousands of people with cancer have used the Bristol Approach to turn the crisis of cancer into an opportunity, and we sincerely hope that this will become possible for you, too.

> The importance of coming to Bristol was the fact that I turned around my whole thought process. I came feeling frightened. I had been told that I had three months to live. The orthodox medicine could do nothing for me and I was just delighted that I could take charge of my own life. I was taught that there were various practices that I could follow – meditation, visualization and relaxation, and a host of other things – and these I followed. It was quite hard in the first place to get into it, but I'm sure they made all the difference to my recovery.
> *Laura Newcombe, living with inoperable bladder cancer, diagnosed in 1985*

The therapies offered at the Centre are discussed in more detail in Chapter 3. The remainder of this chapter outlines the Centre's history, its aims and how its programme works.

An Inspired Idea

The Bristol Cancer Help Centre was the brainchild of acupuncturist Penny Brohn and her close friend Pat Pilkington. Penny was diagnosed with breast cancer in 1979, when she was in her early thirties and had three small children under ten years old. Driven by the imperative to stay alive for them, combined with an acute sense of the inadequacy of the medical model in dealing with both her and her cancer, she set about discovering alternative ways to beat her disease. Strongly encouraged by Pat, she embarked on her healing journey, which was to take her all over the world, inspire the creation of the Bristol Cancer Help Centre, launch her into a media career, and enable her to live with cancer for 20 years from the point of her diagnosis. Her search for alternative medicines that would combat the cancer by strengthening her body's immune system took her first to the metabolic clinic of Dr Josef Issels in Bavaria for immunotherapy. Later she went to the clinic of Dr Ernesto Contreras in Mexico to have metabolic therapy. Back in England, she attended the Mind–Body Centre of Isobel and Maxwell Cade in London, had acupuncture with her long-time mentor Dr Tony Evans, and had spiritual healing with the Reverend Tim Tiley in Bristol. She also visited a remote monastery in the Welsh mountains for meditation retreats.

It was during the nine weeks in Issels' clinic, while undergoing a particularly rigorous treatment, that Penny broke down to Pat, telling her that while she knew this alternative medicine for her body was right, it was really her soul and emotions that were in complete turmoil and desperately needing help. She was terrified of dying, devastated at the thought of leaving her children motherless, and still full of grief having recently lost both parents within weeks of each other. She was also struggling with marital conflicts that had undermined her considerably and left her feeling very isolated.

This sense of isolation was now multiplied a thousandfold as she lay in a German clinic, miles from her family and friends, shivering with fever induced by Dr Issels to boost her immune system. The bottom had completely dropped out of her world. Her wish, which she expressed there and then to Pat, was for a place where all of these treatments and therapies could be brought together under one roof, where body, mind and spirit could be thought about simultaneously – a place under strong medical guidance where all this fear could be contained and all levels of being could be cared for and involved in the process of self-healing.

Pat picked up Penny's thread immediately, asking her how such a centre would be, what it would look like, and what staff and therapies there would be. Fifteen minutes earlier, Penny had been a completely devastated wreck; now, as she built in her mind the ideal centre for people with cancer, she was transformed – absolutely buzzing – as she poured out idea after idea. After about half an hour of this torrent of creativity she suddenly stopped, realized what was happening, and with total conviction said to Pat, 'This is us, Pat, this is what we have got to do. We have to build the Cancer Help Centre.'

As utterly daunting as this felt, with Penny sick and both of them identifying themselves more as housewife than as entrepreneur, they knew immediately that this was it – they would indeed go on to work together to manifest the vision they had created that day. They spent the rest of that week designing and refining their concept. They already had a building, in Downfield Road, Bristol, which Pat and her husband, Canon Christopher Pilkington, had bought to use as a spiritual healing centre. Christopher had latterly spent much of his time developing his ability as a healer under the tutelage of Tim Tiley, and Pat and Penny knew that he would be only too happy to add his support and services to their project. They had friends who were nutritional therapists, so they knew it would be easy to provide expert dietary advice as part of their programme. Counsellors, too, they knew would be no problem to find. The major sticking point was the question of where they would find a doctor in England wanting to work in a holistic way with the treatment of cancer. As Penny said to Pat, 'Why would I be over here in Bavaria miles from my children if there was one single holistic doctor in Britain who was thinking along these lines?'

The First Centre

They came home with this question raging in their minds, only to find that while they had been in Bavaria, Christopher had received a letter from Dr Alec Forbes, a retiring consultant physician who was 'looking for somewhere to put into practice his ideas about the holistic treatment of cancer'. If they had needed any more confirmation that this idea had their names on it, here it was. Very soon Alec was appointed the first Medical Director of the newly named 'Bristol Cancer Help Centre', and they opened on an entirely voluntary basis one day a week at the house in Downfield Road.

Very quickly the news got around, and they were soon full to overflowing with people who were immensely grateful for the support and guidance offered. Word rapidly reached the BBC, and a journalist called Brenda Kidman came to Bristol to make a radio programme called 'The Gentle Path'. She also wrote a book of the same name about her own journey with breast cancer using the Bristol Approach. Several television companies then sent researchers to assess the possibility of making programmes. One young man came down from Glasgow and spent some time mingling with patients and attending group sessions. After a while he came to Pat with tears in his eyes. He confessed that his 'boss' was planning a destructive exposé of the Centre, but he had been so moved by what he had experienced that he couldn't do it. Before he could return with another plan, Penny, Pat and Alec had agreed that the BBC2 *Forty Minutes* team should make a series following the progress of six individuals over a period of about nine months.

The six programmes, called *A Gentle Way with Cancer*, were transmitted in the spring of 1983 and attracted a large audience. The note that had been struck by Penny, Pat, Christopher and Alec resonated deeply with many thousands of people with cancer worldwide, and within weeks the system at Bristol was in complete logjam as demand far exceeded what they could provide. It also became apparent that a day visit to the Centre was not sufficient to enable individuals to cover the ground necessary in order to make the deeper healing changes that are needed to strengthen their chances of recovery. It was now evident that they needed a place where people could stay for a period.

Suddenly they were in the big league, negotiating for large residential premises in the heart of Georgian Clifton. The move to Grove House took place in 1983, and the new Centre was opened on 15 July by His Royal Highness the Prince of Wales, who expressed his wholehearted support for the holistic mind–body–spirit approach to healing that was being promoted by the Centre. With this move came the need to make the transition from being a voluntary organization to being a fundraising charity employing staff to run the expanding therapy programme. However, from this time onwards, those who came to use the Centre were never charged the full cost of the service, all places being subsidized by the charity.

Through the 1980s the Centre flourished, and, as its reputation grew, so did the demand from the media, the public and healthcare professions for education and consultancy services. Help was requested with the design and building of other centres, support groups and hospital-based projects. These enquiries resulted in the setting up of many satellite holistic cancer support groups both in Britain and across the world. Penny and Pat personally helped initiate the establishment of centres in Italy, Sweden, Zimbabwe, South Africa, Hong Kong, Australia, New Zealand, America and Japan. Christopher, meanwhile, took on the role of regularly visiting the 100 or so groups that had sprung up around Britain, helping to encourage, guide and support them in the healing work they were doing.

The most notable of the consultative projects in which the Centre was involved was the Hammersmith Project. This was instigated by Professor Karol Sikora, who had been impressed by the tremendous turnaround he had seen in the morale of his patients who were attending the Centre. He had also observed that some 37 per cent of his patients were already using some form of complementary help or another. After a long period of collaboration, Professor Sikora opened the Hammersmith Hospital Oncology Department Supportive Care Unit in 1991. Here, his department's patients could receive holistic therapies, support and counselling while undergoing conventional treatment for their illness. This unit continues to this day; in 1999 it won the Foundation for Integrated Medicine award for the best model of integrated healthcare practice in Britain.

Troubled Times

However, despite all the very positive progress during the 1980s, there was an undercurrent of antagonism from within the fields of oncology and psycho-social oncology. In a televised discussion following the BBC series *A Gentle Way with Cancer*, Dr Walter Bodmer of the Imperial Cancer Research Fund and Professor Tim McElwain of the Marsden Hospital publicly challenged the heretical assertion being made by Penny and Alec that people with cancer could affect their own prognosis, throwing down the gauntlet that they be allowed to research the Centre's results. In 1984, discussions began and protocols were agreed for the comparison of the survival times and quality of life of two groups of patients with a primary diagnosis of breast cancer: one attending Bristol Cancer Help Centre and a control group of non-attenders.

So, while the Centre's work and reputation were gathering immense momentum, and elsewhere barriers of mistrust within the medical profession were being melted away, the Institute of Cancer Research, funded by the Imperial Cancer Research Fund and Cancer Research Council, was collecting data from Bristol and comparing this information with the Cancer Registry's data on 'matched subjects' who had already died.

In 1990, two years into the five-year trial, the study's director, Professor Claire Chilvers, announced that the interim findings of the study were that people coming to the Centre were relapsing and dying more quickly than people who had had orthodox treatment alone. Rather than investigating these very unlikely statistics further, the cancer charities decided to call an immediate press conference to release these findings. The announcement made the BBC's *Nine O'clock News*, and many thousands of people using the Bristol Approach heard that evening, in this shattering way, that it appeared they were actually putting themselves at serious risk by following the Bristol Approach.

Within days people stopped coming to the Centre; the donors stopped donating, staff were laid off and collapse seemed inevitable. Had the statistics been less dramatic – or even if they had appeared to show that coming to Bristol made no difference at all – the Centre would probably have folded then and there. However, because the findings were so outrageous, many doctors and scientists came to the Centre's rescue, quickly discovering a series of 'fatal flaws' within the study's methodology. It became clear that those who had been studied as 'attenders at the Centre' were a much younger group of women and much more ill than those with whom they had been compared. Also, no check had been made on the extent to which any of these 'Bristol subjects' had fully embarked upon the Bristol Approach: this meant that it was quite possible for somebody who had visited Bristol only once, without ever actually taking up any aspect of the approach, to be counted as a Bristol patient.

The study and its authors were discredited. Tragically, one of the instigators of the study, Professor McElwain, took his own life within weeks of the bitter and vitriolic aftermath of the débâcle. The damage did not stop there. Less than a year after this dreadful fight for the life of the Centre, Penny's own cancer recurred in her spine.

Restoration

The women in the study suffered greatly during the fierce battle between the Centre and the cancer charities. Yet, spearheaded by Heather Goodare and Isla Bourke, they went on to play an extraordinarily heroic role in righting the wrong that had been done to the Centre's reputation, forming the Bristol Survey Support Group. Amazingly, in April 1992 this group managed to get Channel 4 to publicize the story (in a programme called 'Cancer Positive' in the *Free for All* consumer series), and they received apologies from heads of the cancer charities involved. Also in April 1992, they initiated an investigation by the Charities Commission, which in January 1994 found the cancer charities guilty of inadequate supervision of the research.

The Centre will be eternally indebted to these brave women who achieved so much while it clung to the rocks by its fingernails, running a very depleted service with a shoestring staff. During these hard times, major efforts were made to repair the damage to the Centre's credibility and, under the direction of first Dr Michael Weir and then Dr Rosy Daniel, with a team of loyal and experienced therapists, the Centre went on to restore its reputation and, ultimately, to become even stronger than before.

Several factors helped a great deal with this process. First of all, deeply disturbed by the incident and the threat to the Centre's existence, the Prince of Wales gave unstinting support, helping in any way he could to rebuild its network of friends and donors and in 1996 becoming official Patron of the Centre. This vote of confidence gave an enormous boost to the morale of everyone working at the Centre.

The other crucial factor that helped to rebuild the Centre was the rapid evolution of scientific evidence underpinning the approach, most particularly in the newly emerging field of psychoneuroimmunology (PNI),[1] which started to give us an explanation for the mechanism through which both negative and positive emotional influences can affect healing and immune function (see Chapters 2 and 7).

Simultaneously, research evidence was linking diet to cancer, and vitamin and mineral supplementation to cancer prevention. There were also many positive studies on the roles of complementary therapies in improving symptom control, toleration of treatments and the quality of life in people with cancer.

The widespread dissemination of this research work through teaching and media activities during the 1990s led to the making of important documentaries on the role of PNI effects, headed by journalist Alison Delaney in Bristol, and to the inclusion of the Centre's teaching input in the 1998 Annual Conference of the World Health Organization on worldwide cancer strategy. Requests came in for contributions to many of the current teaching textbooks for oncologists. In fact, the Bristol Cancer Help Centre's sphere of influence has become so large in the world of cancer medicine that Professor Karol Sikora, when head of the Cancer Division of the WHO, called it the 'gold standard in complementary cancer care'. The Prince of Wales has described what a 'great pleasure it has been over the years to see how much the Bristol Cancer Help Centre has influenced the development of cancer medicine'.

It is certainly clear from the work of the Prince of Wales Foundation for Integrated Health (initiated by Prince Charles and set up in 1997), which aims to promote the development of integrated medical services in Britain, that far greater progress has been made towards this end in cancer medicine than in any other branch of medicine. It cannot be doubted that a great deal of this progress is owed to the influence of the Bristol Cancer Help Centre.

Penny Brohn's Legacy

Now, at the beginning of the new millennium, the benefits of giving people self-help tools and support to deal with the impact of diagnosis and treatments are being recognized, and complementary supportive care is being incorporated into many cancer units and hospice services. Certainly Penny Brohn never dreamed that within 20 years of the Centre's founding such a level of acceptance and integration would have occurred; and yet, if the present level of momentum and change continues, it seems highly likely that within another ten years people with cancer will be able to experience not only toleration of, but encouragement of, their involvement in their recovery processes.

Penny herself died at home on 3 February 1999 with her now grown-up family around her. She was 'healed into her dying' by two of the Centre's healers, Janet Swan and Cynthia Evanson, and could not have made a more gracious and conscious departure from this world. She proved beyond any shadow of doubt her own complete conviction that cancer is a two-way process over which the individual can have a major influence. During the 20 years she lived after diagnosis, her cancer recurred six times; on each occasion she met the challenge heroically. After reacting each time with entirely appropriate fear and grief, she would come flying back with her own startling creativity, ingenuity, insight and wit, leaving those of us who supported and helped her breathless with admiration.

That Penny should have lived for 20 years with breast cancer is utterly staggering. And Penny's story is only one of the many hundreds of remarkable achievements that have been made by people with cancer who have walked this path in her footsteps. The Bristol Approach to cancer is now her legacy. Her brilliant discoveries, and the many insights and therapeutic developments that have been made over the years at the Centre, continue to be passed on through the work of the expert therapy team and the quite exceptional current therapy programme.

The Centre's Therapeutic Process

The therapeutic process at Bristol Cancer Help Centre has two main aims:

- to help people with cancer to deal with their diagnosis and treatment, and to assist them in finding all possible forms

of medical and complementary support;
- to help promote the health of people with cancer in the presence of their illness.

The first aim, of helping people to deal with the cancer itself, involves giving:

- support and care to help people recover from the diagnosis of cancer (at all stages that cancer is diagnosed);
- medical counselling to help people make difficult medical decisions;
- help in coping with the rigours of treatment;
- help in achieving control of symptoms, both those from the cancer itself and the side-effects of treatment;
- advice about complementary treatments for cancer.

The second aim, of helping to promote health in the presence of illness, is achieved by helping clients to:

- develop a nurturing, responsible and protective relationship with themselves;
- establish healthy eating patterns;
- reduce stress;
- exercise;
- explore personal spirituality;
- attain personal empowerment;
- re-establish meaningful core values;
- realign lifestyle to reflect core values;
- achieve self-expression and promote their own creativity;
- achieve creative, self-expressive, meaningful and purposeful activity.

In practice, these processes go on simultaneously throughout the Centre's programme, and aspects of the two main aims are contained within the roles of all therapists at the Centre.

The Bristol Approach

Getting started on the Centre's therapy programme quite simply involves sending for the self-help pack and booking on one of the courses.

It is helpful to begin the recommended vitamin and mineral regime as soon as you can, rather than waiting until you come to Bristol. It is also a good idea to start addressing the question of changing your diet. To this end you will be helped by *The Healing Foods Cookbook*, by the Centre's Head Chef and Dietary Adviser Jane Sen (see Further Reading, p. 238).

The Bristol Approach is designed for people with cancer and, equally, for those who support them closely. This is because the Approach recognizes that the diagnosis of cancer in a loved one is just as much a life-changing event for the supporter as it is for the person with cancer (see Chapter 8). Therefore all the following descriptions of the courses and their aims apply equally to both people with cancer and their supporters.

The following is an outline of the various components of the programme. Readers should note that, although our philosophy and therapeutic aims remain the same, at times we make small refinements to the content of our courses.

The Self-help Pack
The self-help pack is designed to give you an overall idea of what the Bristol Approach is, and how it might meet your individual needs, so that you can decide whether the therapy programme is suitable for you.

The Two-day Course
Before attending the two-day course you are asked to begin the process of self-evaluation by completing a self-assessment form. This will help you to start thinking about what the key questions and issues are for you so that you

can make the very best use of the time you have with the therapy team at Bristol.

The two-day course is residential. It is very much about meeting others with similar problems, starting the process of recovery from diagnosis, and starting to learn and experience the self-help techniques. On day two, you meet members of the therapy team one-to-one and have in-depth sessions to formulate your own individual assessment and therapy planning process. There will be appointments with the doctor, counsellor, healer and nutritional therapist, and small-group art therapy. By the end of the two days you will have a very clear picture of your therapeutic and self-help needs and will be well and truly embarked on your holistic self-healing journey.

One of the great benefits of embarking on this course is that it enables you to experience solidarity and closeness with others who are going through similar experiences. This plays an important part in helping to achieve many of the course's aims, most especially in reducing the sense of isolation that many people feel after diagnosis. And for the many people who find the idea of making drastic changes in diet quite challenging, the course is especially helpful in that it provides the opportunity for you to discover, by being introduced to organic vegan food, how delicious good, healthy food can be.

The Five-day Course

The aim of the five-day course is to enable people to experience a retreat from everyday life – with plenty of opportunity for reconnection, re-evaluation and renewal. It is a real chance to 'stop the world and get off' for a week, so that you can let go of all your normal considerations – even forgetting that the cancer exists, if that seems possible – in order to get down to the important questions of who you are, and what really matters to you in life.

Some of the questions that the five-day course will encourage you to ask are:

- Where do I wish to put my precious life energy in order to experience the most fulfilment and joy in my life?
- What are my beliefs about living and dying?
- What fears are affecting my life energy, and how can I release these fears?

While this process is going on, your energy will simultaneously be lifted through healing, counselling, massage, shiatsu, meditation, visualization and relaxation. You will also receive advice on your diet and your individual nutritional needs, and there is skilled group facilitation by counsellors, art and music therapists and holistic nurses.

The five-day course is primarily about receiving support and uplift, and taking the time to rest and recover from life's pressures and the difficulties of illness and its treatment, so that you can explore your core values, establish your reason for living, and regain sight of what is important in life. Through this process you can establish your commitment to life or, if appropriate, give yourself permission to let go into your dying process. As you explore yourself and the issues that are relevant to you, you will continue to receive guidance, support and therapy from doctors, nurses and body therapists, and be encouraged to formulate your own self-help plans that will support and stimulate your healing and recovery.

Through learning the skills of healing approaches, which include personal imagery and affirmation, you will increase your understanding of the role of the mind in affecting the physiology of the body, and future life and illness outcomes. You will continue to learn the self-help techniques of meditation, visualization and relaxation, and to form a healthy eating plan, strengthening your body through excellent food, exercise, stretching and breathwork. In doing this you will increase your awareness of the body's energy state, and learn the skills to improve this on a day-to-day basis.

The five-day course can be an intense experience, in that it provides you with the support that enables you to journey into your pain, to express profound and difficult emotions, to face your fear, losses, disability, despair and anger and, if you wish, to face death itself. This chance to air the unspeakable often liberates a great deal of trapped energy, which can lead to an enormous sense of relief and renewed vitality.

Through these processes you will be able to focus on the positive side of your experience of illness, enabling you to:

- work through and resolve the negative emotions and situations that block your life and healing;
- look at the possible secondary gains of the illness, and learn how to get the same benefits in healthy ways;
- look at the message the cancer may be giving you;
- experience creativity and self-expression through art, music and movement;
- become 'true to yourself' by becoming more aware of your feelings;
- become bolder and clearer in communicating your needs to others (for some people this may involve assertiveness training) and more authentic in the way you make your day-to-day and life choices.

What the Five-day Course has Meant to Participants

We have lost count of the number of people who have said to us that the week at the Bristol Cancer Help Centre was the best week of their lives. Indeed, many have said that everyone should go through this programme – regardless of whether or not they have cancer – so that they can look at how they are living, shed their fears and learn to express themselves and their potential fully.

The changes people go through during the week range from being very practical and outwardly focused to very profound and more to do with the inner state of being. Whichever they are, people almost always leave the five-day course deeply heartened by the experience and the loving support and encouragement they have felt during their visit.

The extremely potent atmosphere that exists during this course is created through the mutual bonding of the members of the group who attend, and the highly individualized care given by the multidisciplinary team of holistic therapists who meet two to three times a day to give each other constant feedback on the evolving needs and state of all participants as the process unfolds. Of course, the most basic ingredients are a combination of the Centre's healing environment (which feels safe enough for individuals to embark upon a deep self-healing journey) and the strong belief, held by all who work at the Centre, that remarkable recovery and healing of spirit, mind and body are possible. What we never know is who will recover, to what degree and at what level the greatest healing changes will occur. It is always apparent, however, that if the spirit is lifted and healed, the individual is enabled both to live and to die immeasurably more comfortably and happily.

It is clear that the road to healing is a very personal one, and it therefore differs from person to person, but for all there is great delight in learning to be guided by their own wisdom and intuition. This sense of unfolding discovery has been described by many as a terrifically exciting adventure, and the deeper sense that is often created in the individual during the process might be called one of 'finally coming home to oneself'. This has been described by others as moving out of their false self, in other words discarding learned patterns and ways of being, and shedding the defences that kept them locked in unhappy, limited lives.

It is as if, having been cracked open by the fear of the diagnosis, all the smaller fears that have been limiting life implode. Given the presence of a great deal of unconditional healing, love and encouragement, astounding transformational change can occur, bringing people into a completely different relationship with themselves, both in their living and in their dying. As the spirit is healed or lifted there is often a growing memory or awareness that in fact death itself is not so frightening after all and, as this process deepens, the sense of inner strength and personal authority grows.

With this growing awareness, the resistance to change melts, while at the same time there is a paradoxical increase in the sense of control. This might be likened to the feeling you experience when you first succeed at riding a bicycle. As impossible and improbable as it felt the day before when you were unable to do it, you are now able to hold this dynamic balance and enjoy the great new freedom that it gives you.

The Follow-up Day

The follow-up day is a one-day course that can be undertaken at any time after attending either of the residential courses.

The day starts with a group meeting, first to relax and then to share together the roller-coaster of life and the healing process since the last visit. One of the great pleasures of this day is that newcomers meet the inspiring people who have been coming to the Centre for years and will witness the marvellous example that they set: as many of these people say, 'I should have been dead years ago.'

This introductory group is followed by one-to-one sessions with the doctor, healer, nutritional therapist and counsellor, and art therapy in small groups. At the end of the day there is another discussion forum to reflect on the progress made and to troubleshoot any outstanding problems.

The Follow-up Nurse

It must be acknowledged that the process that the Centre is offering to its clients is a complex and demanding one. Essentially, it involves the taking on board of a new model of healthcare before starting, and choosing among and embarking upon many new practices and therapies.

The benefits of the Bristol Approach
Over 20 years, observation of the Bristol Approach and feed-back from patients indicate that receiving loving support and embracing the holistic approach can bring extremely positive benefits to physical, emotional and spiritual well-being, by:

- reducing fear – achieving a calm, balanced, happy state of mind through healing massage, relaxation and counselling;
- strengthening the body – through stress reduction, healthy eating, vitamin and mineral supplementation, and physical exercise such as yoga, tai chi and chi gong;
- raising your energy – through spiritual healing, bodywork and creative self-expression;
- healing the heart – by letting go of past hurts and disappointment, and by learning to express emotion, improve communication and become true to yourself;
- changing your mind – replacing limiting or unhealthy attitudes or beliefs with very strongly life-affirming messages, images and goals;
- lifting the spirit – by focusing on what gives you joy, fulfilment, purpose and meaning in your life;
- enhancing your life – building a healthy, fulfilling lifestyle around your newly prioritized values and sources of nourishment.

In order to maintain the programme that you have created through your visits to the Centre, it is very important that in the early stages assistance and support are available to help you make the right contacts in the home environment. To this end the follow-up nurse will phone clients between courses to give the necessary guidance and encouragement, and generally hear how things are going. This feedback enables the Centre to determine the extent to which people continue to implement the Bristol Approach once they get back home and are subjected to the old pressures and the expectations of others; in addition, it provides valuable information about the quality of the courses and the clients' reaction to them.

Who Will Benefit from the Bristol Approach?

The Bristol Approach is unique in Britain, and almost unique in the world, in offering in-depth mind–body medicine. The approach improves the ability to cope with the diagnosis and treatment of cancer, and ultimately can turn the crisis of cancer into the opportunity for living far more happily and healthily than before. The Bristol Approach has a great deal to offer anyone, but it is especially important for those who feel that their spirit has been crushed by difficult and painful life events, or who have lost their way in life, or who recognize themselves as self-stressors or workaholics, or who are aware that their energy levels or mood are low, or that in one way or another they do not take very good care of their health.

Not all aspects of the Bristol Approach will be right for everyone, but usually the obvious starting point will become clear quickly, and it may be that over time your use of the approach will increase as you explore it further – a bit like peeling the different layers from an onion. For example, over four years in her recovery from the treatment for secondary ovarian cancer, Sarah Hughes of Bristol tackled first her nutrition and physical health. In year two she moved, having initially resisted it, into counselling, unburdening herself of the considerable emotional distress she was carrying; in year three she used energy medicines, which significantly enhanced her level of health, and, in year four, she was able to embrace her spirituality by joining the Quakers and thus finally to put the whole jigsaw together.

2
Science and the Bristol Approach

David Beales

This chapter explores the Bristol Approach in relation to the 'biomedical' model of established medical practice and shows how it can be beneficially combined with conventional treatment and care. David Beales is a retired GP and has a longstanding interest in mind–body medicine. He is a member of the BCHC therapy advisory board.

Integrative Medicine: Towards a Whole-Person Approach

The previous chapter emphasized that the Bristol Approach by no means excludes recourse to orthodox medical treatment and care, and that most people who come to the Centre opt for some balance of the orthodox medical and holistic/complementary routes. However, it is also important to stress that the treatment and care offered by the Centre are founded on principles that extend beyond the usual concerns of established modern medicine to address the whole person and his or her life.

The Bristol Approach considers the whole person. In other words, we view each individual's health, or illness, as resulting from all the many interacting influences on body, mind and spirit. This involves reviewing, among other factors, the influence of our environment and of the communities in which we live. As we step back and look at our situation in the round, we can see the impact of the complex pressures working on and through us. This more complete picture is central to our approach. It allows us to tease out the path that will allow each individual to find his or her way forward with a strengthened and well-functioning immune system, so that the whole person – mind, body and spirit – is primed for recovery and well-being.

Our approach contrasts with the conventional model of medicine that prevails in the West today. In this view, often called the 'biomedical' approach, the body is seen as a machine, and an illness or disease, such as cancer, as the result of a malfunction in the machine. According to this model, disease is a specific fault that can be remedied by correcting that fault. This leads logically to the dominant position of surgery, radiotherapy, chemotherapy and other modern conventional treatments in the treatment of cancer.

It is important to remember that cancer is an extremely complicated disease with multiple causes and influences – genetic, environmental, nutritional, stress-related, etc. The Bristol Approach involves looking at all the possible interactions fostering disease, and also the personal circumstances in which the illness has arisen. Of course, there are complex local factors, involving tissues, cells, the immune system and chemistry, producing a cancer at the cellular level; but in our view that is not the whole story. To concentrate wholly on these local physical aspects and ignore what is happening to the person as a whole is to fail to understand the profound way in which we are interconnected with each other and all that is around us.

The problem with the conventional or biomedical model is that, although resulting in wonderful scientific discoveries that have made possible technical advances in treatment, it tends to create a culture in which the individual may feel estranged from fellow human beings, overwhelmed by the technology, without control and fearful.

It is, we believe, when the individual *both* feels genuinely involved in taking and implementing the decisions surrounding his or her own treatment and care, *and* is able to take advantage of the best of medical scientific progress that he or she has the best chance of regaining health and well-being. In pursuit of this ideal combination, the Bristol Approach allows the individual to:

- step back from the immediate pressures of his or her situation, in a uniquely nurturing and sustainable environment;
- look at his or her needs for both the present and the future;
- create a restorative plan; and
- work in partnership with conventional professional advisers.[2]

The Scientific Evidence

What is the evidence that getting involved with our health makes any difference to the quality of our life, let alone our very survival? The answer to the first part of the question is clear. Where people actively work with their medical team in a partnership approach, anxiety and depression levels fall markedly. Professor Leslie Walker,[3] who now runs a cancer health centre in Hull, showed this clearly in the cancer care service at Aberdeen, where people had access to advice on all aspects of the conventional medical treatment, together with encouragement, for those who were interested, to take up and use such techniques such as relaxation, hypnosis and guided imagery. Indicators of significant anxiety and distress among those treated fell from, on average, 30 per cent for those who were not offered the additional techniques to the order of 5 per cent for those who were.

Alastair Cunningham,[4] a senior research scientist at the Ontario Cancer Institute in Canada, summarizing the research evidence, noted that substantial improvements in quality of life (e.g. less anxiety and depression, more sense of control, better communication with other people) follow the approaches outlined in this chapter. He also confirms that there is a growing body of evidence, which his unit's clinical experience supports, that psychological self-help work can not only prolong life but also bring about unexpected remission in some cases. So, getting involved with your own health can actually influence your survival as well as the quality of your life.

Our Human Needs

Each person has human needs that have evolved over the lifetime of our species. The increasing complexity of our Western materialistic lifestyle puts increasing pressure on the individual's resources, and may lead to the neglect of these essential human requirements.

What are the essential human needs?[5] Academic researchers have identified among them a list that is shown in the box on page 27. Clearly, the pursuit, fulfilment and/or denial of these needs brings into our lives such additional factors as happiness, anger and sustained stress, anxiety and depression, and the capacity for humour.

Just as much as we all share certain common needs, so these take particular form in each person's own life and circumstances. In the Bristol Approach we start from the perspective that each person is – or can be – the greatest expert on himself or herself. We acknowledge that many important

---

The core human needs
- autonomy and control;
- connection to others;
- purpose and goals;
- spiritual connection;
- mind–body understanding;
- creativity;
- giving and receiving attention.

---

factors affecting health are within the individual's control. Our aim is to enable individuals with cancer to become aware of the state of their lives – their bodies, minds and spirit – in order to create planned restoration and a rebalancing process. One of the first stages in this process is for each individual to be able to identify his or her own particular needs, recognize that they are legitimate and learn how best to meet them. One way to set about this is to ask yourself the following questions.

Attitudes of mind
- Is there a balance in my life between time for myself and time I give to others, or do I put everyone else first?
- Do I have a free choice in my life, or do I constrict and limit my life and energy by dictating to myself what I 'ought' and 'ought not' to do?
- Is there a balance in my life between work and play, or am I a 'workaholic'?
- Am I comfortable asking for help?

What place do feelings and emotions have in my life?
- In general, do I easily express my feelings, or keep a 'stiff upper lip'?
- Can I risk saying what I feel, speaking my own truth, even if it makes me unpopular in others' eyes?

Creative potential
- What abilities or attributes do I value in myself? Can I name three?
- Has my capacity for play, for experiencing personal pleasure, increased or decreased in recent years?
- If I take a moment or two to recall joyous times in my life, what do they have in common?
- What is a source of joy in my life now, and what might be a source of joy in the future?

The spiritual self
- Do I have a sense that there is a divine part in us all, seeking us?
- Do I have a sense of an energy that is both internal and external to my body?
- Where do I feel close to such an energy, e.g. in nature, beauty, work, creativity . . . ?

Early Influences and the 'False Self'

High on the list of human needs identified above is that for 'connection with others' – experienced by most of us as the need for love and approval. The restoration of health is thus likely to involve looking at how we have – or have not – met this need. For many, this exploration will lead on to transforming low self-worth and a poor self-image into a state of positive self-worth with a positive sense of self – and to doing this without blaming others.

Our personality and sense of self develop from childhood, on two levels: first, from our genetic inheritance, via our parents; and second, through our own unique experiences within our particular environment – in families, communities, schools and so on. The individual's unique personality evolves in response to how the environment acts on the hereditary material. If we grow up with a positive, appreciative attitude around us, this encourages a sense of worth, creating a strong sense of self and the ability to love ourselves, together with an ability to recognize, reach towards and attain our human needs. However, if we have grown up with negative feedback and a lack of appreciation, this fosters a low sense of self-worth and a poor self-image. By adulthood this pattern of thinking has become subconscious and automatic – and hard to relinquish. Indeed, the self tends to hold on to this lack of self-worth. It has become like a well-worn coat: comfortable and safe, even if it lets in the rain now and again. Thus any attempt to overturn the established patterning is likely to be resisted.

Sometimes we are aware of these influences, but sometimes there is a discrepancy between how we consciously see our lives and the buried emotional reaction to negative experience, which is not available to us. Lydia Temoschok has described in her researches how this creates a helpful exterior,[6] while inwardly the individual is hurting. At the Bristol Cancer Help Centre, we see it as hugely important to address these issues, for we know, from this researcher and others cited later in this chapter, that depression, hopelessness and despair are associated with the poorest outcomes among people with cancer. Discovering the subconscious pattern and working to overcome the ingrained 'false self' requires the assistance of skilled counselling; particularly appropriate is transpersonal therapy, described in more detail elsewhere in this book (see pp. 62–6).

Starting from Now – Looking to the Future

Reconnection with the genuine self and the restoration of self-esteem is a prominent part of the whole-person approach. A positive self-image means developing a caring and tender relationship with yourself. Often this means learning simply to say 'no' to the demands and expectations of others. At the same time, inherent in the new relationship with the self that we are

---

The lone flower

A once-beautiful flower, struggling with its health, found it difficult to hold up its heavy bloom and to let the sun in. So it closed its petals and let its head droop forward; and it stopped trying to push its roots deep into the soil. Without a daily renewal of life force, it felt old beyond its time and very tired.

But then . . . slowly the flower began to relax its tissues, gently allowing in the nutrients from the soil and the healing warmth from the sun. As it did so, its slumped stem began to straighten and its downward gaze began to lift.

One day the flower stretched with all its might and was able to hold its bloom fully upright once again. To its delight, when it looked up and around the flower realized that it wasn't alone . . . but was in a beautiful garden with other flowers and plants at different stages of growth. At that moment the numbness left its contracted roots and this once withering flower stood tall, as it savoured the sensations of feeling its roots intertwined with those of various other plants around it. Now it basked in the warmth of the sun and realized that it was not isolated but deeply connected to all the other living things in the garden. Thus a blessing was given to the flower that had the courage to open up and give life a second chance, in order to rediscover its own special place in the garden of life.

---

trying to nurture is the giving up of the passive assumption that we can expect others to put things right. All of us, while we should be aware of the past and how it has shaped us, have to start from where we are now, beginning without any unhelpful self-judgement.

Let us take the analogy of a property where the garden has been neglected for many years. Instead of bringing in outside experts straight away, the first thing to do is to see the weeds and the flowers, to choose what to preserve, and to remove those that are choking what may be waiting to bloom underneath. Then, instead of digging everything up, we will wait to see what new life is going to emerge. The nurturing of the new life as it appears is exciting, and we encourage it with light, nutrients and care. After a year or so we may want to move plants, add new ones, change the layout, create more interest and excitement. The first stage, however, is one of patient anticipation of good things to come. The box on page 30, 'The lone flower', develops a metaphor which some have found useful.

So, in the Bristol Approach, we see moving towards and promoting health and well-being as a three-stage process:

1   Look at your life and see what aspects may be choking your life force and draining your energy, overburdening, depressing or overloading you. Sometimes it is necessary to find a guide, ideally a counsellor trained in appropriate therapy, to help you look for and identify the weeds. Prepare for new growth.
2   Gently identify and remove those 'weeds' that are no longer serving you in your evolution and renewal.
3   Look for the emerging life force and energy, nourishing and encouraging your new aliveness.

Dealing with Depression

One of the potential pitfalls in this approach that needs to be considered is the possibility that, faced with this newly diagnosed threat to life, you have responded with depression. This is a very understandable response, but gets in the way of recovery as it leads to neglect of your own needs and to 'black and white' thinking – seeing everything other than total success as complete failure – and thus to difficulty in seeing that recovery is possible even in the face of life-threatening diagnosis.

The Bristol Approach involves recognizing and nurturing those parts of ourselves that are absolutely fine, and just need a little of the light of day to thrive.

Ask yourself these questions:

•   Over the past two weeks, have I felt down, depressed or hopeless?

31

- Over the past two weeks, have I felt little interest or pleasure in doing things?

If the answer to either question is 'yes', then your first priority must be to move out of this state – to lift yourself out of the sense of hopelessness and helplessness that is the major component of depression.

Research has shown that counselling is able to lift people out of hopeless and helpless states. Counselling can enable you to look afresh at your predicament – at which point people usually find that they have strengths and past achievements that they can use again to help them recover from the diagnosis of cancer.

Taking Control

It often happens, that, having inwardly begun to take control in the way suggested above, people become more assertive in their dealings with medical professionals and institutions. Doctors do not always welcome this; but it is a positive development, for an active partnership creates not only autonomy but also genuine cooperative working. In this process it may be necessary to choose carefully the team of health professionals involved with your treatment. Do they involve you in seeking an effective partnership with them? It is vital that you put yourself and your needs first – that you become 'full of self'.

I was devastated by the secondary diagnosis – completely destroyed. I went through the conventional treatment very successfully but realized this was a warning I could not ignore. I needed to take a long hard look at my lifestyle – the hours I was working, the stress of my job, the lack of sleep, and the junk food – and make some dramatic changes for the future.
Angela Burns, living with secondary breast cancer, first diagnosed in 1991

Learning to Listen to Yourself

All of us have a great deal of information available to ourselves, through an inner voice that can be a wise guide when we quieten down enough to hear it. This inner voice can be lost when we lose our own authenticity, our genuine self, and act on the basis of what we think others expect of us. Several therapies used in the Bristol Approach, and described in more detail in the next chapter, work towards allowing this inner voice, this intuitive sense of self, to become audible. It often becomes reconnected in meditation, when the busy mind becomes calm and a sense of real needs emerges. Guided imagery,[7] too, can greatly help in finding our own wise guide and inner healing capacity. We can also reconnect with the inner needs when they appear in symbols and dreams; art therapies can help us tap into this inner language. The skill of transpersonal counselling is also particularly refined to enable us to understand the language of our inner voice. In all these ways we aim to restore the balance between the various elements of the personality and the psyche.

> I discovered an inner life that I certainly didn't know I had, and certainly wasn't nurturing, and I discovered how valuable and healing that was. I learned to be still and listen to my body's needs. I changed my life quite radically. I have given up full-time work (and am fortunate in being able to do a variety of paid and unpaid part-time work). I have more leisure time – and a lot more fun!
> *Angela Burns, living with secondary breast cancer, first diagnosed in 1991*

Regaining a Healing Metabolism

When we are looking after ourselves, in the full sense, we find we are naturally taking care of good nutritional and physical

Anger/guilt/negative emotions

Persistent stress/over-arousal

Poor sleep

Depression/despair/hopelessness

Leading to:

Diminished sense of control with

Altered and deregulated physiology

Catabolic metabolism

Cortisol levels often raised

Immune depression

Fig. 1: The influence of over-stimulation of internal systems on our bodies

fitness. With this we will find that the body regulates itself and we sleep well, breathe easily and have enough energy for our essential needs. On the other hand, when we are not taking full care of ourselves, or when we are chronically stressed, the body responds in ways that we need to learn to recognize.

Figure 1 summarizes the influence of emotions and stress on

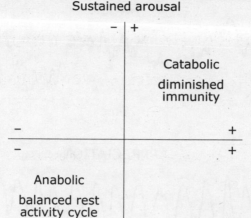

Fig. 2: *Henry's 'axis' diagram: anabolic and catabolic metabolism (after the originator, Jim Henry)*

our body metabolism. When we are under long-term stress, that part of the nervous system that works automatically to regulate functions like the circulation of the blood and the production of hormones, as well as 'chemical messengers' associated with negative emotion (we will learn more of these 'chemical messengers' later in this chapter) becomes too dominant. Our 'drive system' overheats.

When a cancer has developed, the body may have got used to this particular internal state, which in popular terms we might call 'overdriven' or 'overstressed', and which in medical jargon is called a 'catabolic metabolism'. Here the internal chemistry has reacted to sustained overload, and the first essential for healing is to restore the metabolism to one that is self-regulating and in balance. This metabolism is called 'anabolic', and is the metabolism that is associated with health rather than

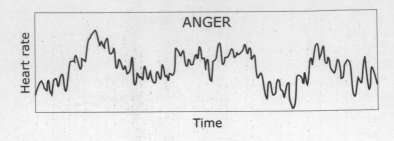

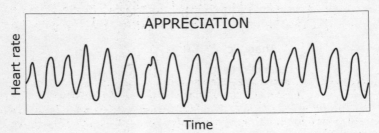

Fig. 3: (a, top) Negative emotion and heart rate variability; (b, above) positive emotion and heart rate variability (© copyright 2001, Institute of HeartMath)

illness. To help rebalance the system and return the metabolism to an anabolic state, therapies that reduce the dominance of the automatic nervous system, such as massage, reflexology, and various body therapies such as shiatsu, yoga and craniosacral osteopathy, as well as healing, are likely to be beneficial.

When we are in the overdriven, 'catabolic' state, different elements of our body system may show the strain: for example, we might develop high blood pressure, or a depressed and less efficient immune system. Sustained negative emotion, such as fear or anger, has a destabilizing effect on the ability of the body's systems to regulate themselves and to relate to one another in a sustainable and balanced way.

We can see the effect of this overdriven, exhausted metabolism on internal systems by monitoring core body functions

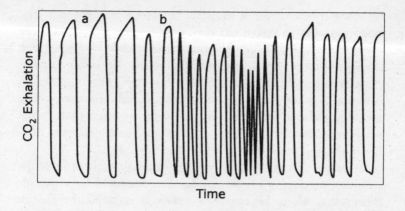

Fig. 4: Capnogram showing drop in a 36-year-old male patient's end tidal CO_2 while relaxing (a), and starting to think (with frustration) about a missed job promotion (b). Trace duration was 90 seconds. Each wave represents a breath: peaks are end points of breathing out. (Reproduced from Multidisciplinary Approaches to Breathing Pattern Disorders, Churchill Livingstone, *2002, with permission from Elsevier Science.)*

such as heartbeat and breathing. The beat-to-beat variation in the heart rate, instead of responding to fluctuations in internal body rhythms with a self-regulating, flexible pattern, tends instead to lack flexibility in its pattern. Figure 3(a) shows the disorganized rhythm produced in conditions of strong negative emotion and, for comparison, Figure 3(b) shows the synchronized heart wave of health – called coherence.

The normal breathing patterns that maintain the chemistry of body systems in a state of balance are also likely to be disturbed. When the natural and normal breathing reflex of quiet abdominal breathing is overridden by chronic arousal (as in Figure 4, which shows the effect of frustration on the exhalation of carbon dioxide), the body's carbon dioxide is reduced, causing profound metabolic changes. When carbon dioxide exhalation is increased by hyperventilation or 'overbreathing', an overall lack of carbon dioxide develops which indirectly means that less oxygen is available to meet essential needs. The body then has to resort to other mechanisms to maintain the essential balance between alkalinity and acidity. Overbreathing causes the blood to become too alkaline; so, in order to compensate, the body 'dumps' alkalis in the urine, accompanied by essential minerals such as magnesium and potassium. The resulting deficits within the body are thought to result in the widespread bodily symptoms, such as weakness, dizziness, tingling and chest pain, that go with overbreathing.

As many as a third of the population may overbreathe to the extent of producing a breathing pattern disorder.[8] Certainly for asthmatics, when the breathing reflex is restored there is an accompanying restoration of the quality of life and a decrease in asthma severity.[9]

At the Bristol Cancer Help Centre, people can be guided to see whether they are overbreathing and are given support in returning breathing to a balanced state. A screening questionnaire, validated by research to identify the overbreathing pattern – the 'Nijmegen questionnaire' – gives a good idea whether chronic overbreathing is a problem, in which case the individual may be recommended to take up a breathing retraining programme.

I was bottling everything up all the time, and then finally I realized that this was one of my biggest problems, and it was causing me a lot of trouble. I found different ways to release all this tension, and the first obvious thing was to have a good cry – it was amazing how good it made me feel afterwards. The other thing I found was singing at the top of my voice in the car (which I never used to do) – and I've got a terrible voice! I just felt more and more relaxed as time went on, and felt much better in myself.

Reg Flower, living with secondary melanoma, first diagnosed in 1981

Energy and Life Force

The concept of energy is central to the ancient models of health maintenance from the East. Within China's 5,000-year-old medical tradition, this fundamental energy is called *chi*, and Chinese medical treatment (including acupuncture) aims at rebalancing the energy channels or meridians. Similarly, in Japan, shiatsu works towards the restoration of *ki*. In the Indian yogic tradition, energy is called *prana*; in the West we might call it *joie de vivre*. In all these cultures, the state of underlying energy is central to the well-being of the whole organism.

Energy and Balance

Let us look now at where energy is placed. How do you allocate it among the different aspects of your life: work, the home, family and friends, spouse or partner – and yourself? If you give yourself a hundred units to represent all the energy you have in, say, an average week, and divide them up among these categories, you will get an idea of where your energy goes. Is most of it spent in one area? How many points did you allocate to 'yourself'?

In looking at our relationships with ourselves, with others and with life itself, the emphasis is on seeking to achieve equilibrium, the right balance for you. The Chinese describe this as a state of balance between the forces of yin (representing what we call the 'dominant sympathetic drive' of the automatic nervous system) and yang (representing the qualities associated with calm and relaxation) – a state of harmony. With the achievement of harmony comes a sense of the interconnectedness of life, an increased sense of inner knowing, with enhanced personal intuition and understanding.

Ten years ago perhaps it was the material things that were of value to me – power of impression, prestige. But nowadays it is my close friends, it is nature (I find a lot of strength in nature), it's my family. We live in the woods, and I don't have a rush, rush, rush lifestyle as I did previously. I think it has been very healing.

Zoe Lindegrin, living with lung secondaries from breast cancer, first diagnosed in 1988

Making Time for Yourself: Facing Fears

In order to make time for ourselves, we need also to ask how the energies of other people may affect us. If you are somebody who tends to care for others and to watch out for their comfort rather than your own needs, it is possible that you may take on or soak up the difficult energies of others. An environment of harmony and peace need not be obtained at the expense of looking after yourself; let your own needs become paramount as you take charge and develop your health recovery plan.

Think again about where energy has tended to concentrate by looking once more at the number of units you allocated to each area of your life. Do you find that time for self is displaced by overwork? Or chronic busyness? Perhaps in overgiving? There is often a pressing need to timetable space for ourselves into our lifestyle. Time for the individual, alone, is important so that we can become aware of what has been happening to us. The aim is to look freshly with our observing self and to conserve our energy so that healing begins and is sustained.

It may be that you will feel resistance and anger building as you read these sentences. 'How can I change what is expected of me?' you may ask; 'I have my duties and obligations.' It is possible that such resistance to the idea of being alone may be prompted by unconscious reminders of previous periods of distress, loneliness and fear. Many people fear that the moment they stop doing or focusing on outward activities, life may become unbearable. If so, then a counsellor can help us negotiate a way into our silent inner space, and to create a new relationship with our inner self that will begin a process of self-nurture. Through this means, too, we also often find a reconnection with our spiritual core; meditators describe this

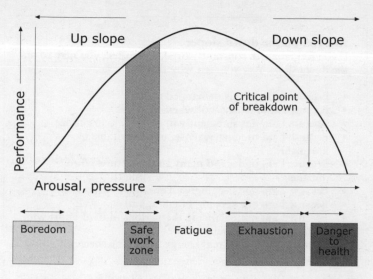

Fig. 5: Pressure and fatigue: the human function curve (after Nixon)

state as one of connection with the divine, or a state of non-duality. Similar submerged feelings can also block meditation, when we are alone with ourselves; however, meditation can allow us to come face to face with these very fears in a safe environment in such a way that they are simply allowed to rise up and fall away, with the inner knowing that 'this too will pass'.

The availability of a retreat away from everyday pressures becomes vital for many in this process. To provide such a place of refuge is a vital aspect of the therapeutic healing environment at the Bristol Cancer Help Centre, where great emphasis is placed on beauty, contact with nature, sustainable living, tranquillity, comfort, and emotional and spiritual safety. People coming to the Centre often remark on these qualities when entering the space.

Energy and Fatigue
As human beings, we respond well to pressure – up to a point.

41

Are you on the down slope?
If you feel fatigued, constantly tired, exhausted, you may be on the down slope. Ask yourself why this might be.

- Because too much is demanded of me?
- Because I cannot say 'no' when needed?
- Because I am not sufficiently in control? Can't cope?
- Because I am too angry, tense, upset, irritable or indignant?
- Because I am under too many time pressures? Too impatient?
- Because I am not sleeping well enough to keep well?
- Because I am not keeping fit enough to stay well?
- Because I am not balancing the periods of hard effort with adequate sleep and relaxation?
- Because I am out of real energy and using sheer willpower to keep going?

But so often, that point is passed without our realizing it, and healthy activity becomes unsustainable pressure. The human function curve (Figure 5) shows how too much pressure gives rise to fatigue and then exhaustion. If we push ourselves too hard over time, we pass our peak performance and move over the top and into the down slope of the curve. Too much has been demanded of us to maintain our health, and the 'over-driven' catabolic metabolism results.

Initially we feel tiredness and then persistent fatigue; this is the body's way of telling us to draw back, restore and re-energize. Figure 6(a–c) shows how energy levels change over time and changing circumstances.

Low Energy Levels
Together, Figures 5 and 6 give us a picture of what happens when energy levels fall below a comfortable and sustainable level for the individual. This applies not only to people with cancer or

The protesting body
If you are fatigued, your body is trying to tell you something.
Ask yourself:

- What is it trying to say?
- Am I listening?
- Why is it protesting?
- Am I able to work to make it stronger or am I too upset with myself to succeed?

other health problems, but also to those who look after them. We know from research that when carers are overloaded,[10] not only do they become susceptible to colds and minor ailments, but also they cease to be able to respond with antibodies when given an influenza vaccine. In other words, their immune system is working less well than it should be. When an individual reaches his or her own critical point on the down slope of the human function curve, the immune system is seriously underactive.

It is at this point that the SABRES model (see Figure 7) can help. Reappraising your life at this stage may be too much of a challenge; rest and restoration of the metabolism must be the priorities. A person faced with the diagnosis of cancer, with a likely further increase in stress (arousal in the figure), often precipitated by the haste with which conventional treatment is presented, may be exhausted. It would be dangerous at this point to add to the load by asking for a complete reappraisal of lifestyle, intensive meditation and/or visualization – and a total change of diet may be the final straw! Most crucially of all, low energy levels can engender demotivation and even loss of the will to live. In this depleted state, self-help becomes almost completely impossible or, worse still, counterproductive.

Clearly, then, it is vitally important to make an accurate assessment of current energy levels. Often in the midst of illness our energy levels are low. This happens because we have been in

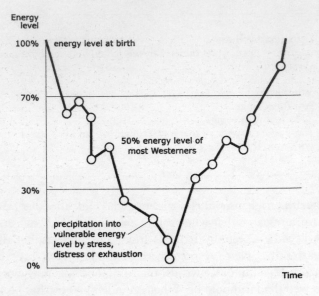

energy level at birth

50% energy level of most Westerners

precipitation into vulnerable energy level by stress, distress or exhaustion

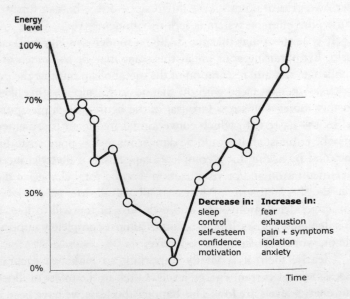

Decrease in:
sleep
control
self-esteem
confidence
motivation

Increase in:
fear
exhaustion
pain + symptoms
isolation
anxiety

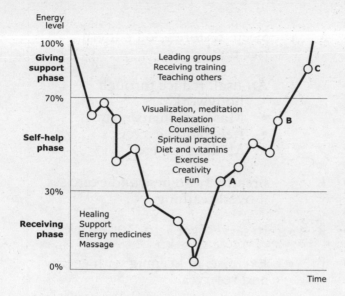

At point C, energy is sufficient for the individual to offer help and support to others

At point B, self-help has succeeded in raising energy to above the normal level for most Westerners

At point A, the energy level has been raised sufficiently for self-help to begin

Fig. 6: Energy levels. (a, top left) The energy model: energy plummets as health deteriorates, and rises again as health is improved through therapy and self-help. (b, bottom left) The effect on the individual's state of mind when energy level falls below the critical 30% level. (c, above) The phases of recovery. When energy is below the critical 30% level, therapy is necessary for the process of recovery to begin. Self-help must then be instigated to ensure that energy does not fall back below the critical level, and that the recovery process continues.

- S : Sleep: restore good pattern
         (see text)

- A : Arousal: reduce through
         - Bodywork
         - Massage, shiatsu, etc.
         - Relaxation exercises
         - Meditation, etc.

- B : Breath: awareness and exercises
         if overbreathing

- R : Reserves: keep 20–30% back

- E : Exercise: in keeping with energy
         and reserves

- S : Self-esteem returns

Fig. 7: The SABRES model: sleep, arousal, breath, reserves, exercise, self-esteem (after Nixon)

a state of struggle. To self-assess your current state of energy, give yourself time to reflect inwardly on where you would place your energy level on a scale of 1 to 10, where 10 is the most energized you could feel. If you put your current energy level at 3 or below, you will need to focus initially on a sleep, rest and restoration programme,[11] with the emphasis on the body and touch therapies. Finding a place of safety away from the demands of everyday life, and where care is offered with unconditional love, becomes a prerequisite until energy levels have been restored to the upward slope of the human function curve.

Restoring Energy Levels

At the Centre, therapies that have been found to increase energy include spiritual healing, the body therapies of shiatsu and acupuncture, and massage and aromatherapy. Contact with a good therapist also reduces fear. Any therapeutic session where relaxation is induced allows the individual to recognize the mind–body connection leading to the relaxed state, and in time, as energy levels return to an adequate level, he or she can begin to learn self-help techniques.

When people have very low energy levels it is necessary for them to receive help, and to let go. This is difficult for many people who find it hard to relinquish control – in other words, people who always give rather than take. Also, when energy levels begin to rise, people who have not been aware of the mechanisms that caused the previous patterns of overload tend to want to return to old lifestyles and patterns of behaviour. It is at this point that intervention to introduce new patterns of thinking and living becomes timely.

For individuals with a cancer diagnosis, it is usually possible to negotiate time to put themselves first. This next phase of self-help will probably focus on developing a plan that is likely to involve the exploration of new behaviours, perhaps with a counsellor, engaging in strategies to restore hope, and finding a spiritual practice that is right for the individual. There will usually be a focus on a healthy diet and relaxation techniques; meditation and visualization may be introduced for those who choose to add these elements to their recovery plan. The creative therapies – art therapy, dance, creative writing – can also be very valuable, and a narrative diary in which you record your experiences, both negative and positive, is likely to prove therapeutic. Gentle exercise, possibly including yoga or tai chi, can be introduced. (Again, all these therapies are described in more detail in Chapter 3.)

Through this plan, and all the various therapies, activities and strategies it involves, you establish a different sort of

An exercise to raise energy and release tension

Dr Jim Gordon, the founder of the Centre for Mind–Body Medicine, recommends starting the day with a favourite piece of lively music and dancing along with it. This awakening and rebalancing exercise might also be included in the 20-minute break between 90-minute cycles of activity during the day. The method he suggests is as follows:

- Plant your feet solidly on the ground. Let your arms hang loosely at your sides, and make sure that your knees are bent. Let your body become loose as you begin to shake, or bounce your entire body up and down, keeping your feet planted. Drop your jaw; let your head rest easily on your neck. Let your body make what ever sound it wants to make. Continue for about 5–10 minutes.
- Turn on the dance music, and let yourself move freely in whatever way feels right.

Be sure to stay within your capacity, holding enough in reserve to remain comfortable and able to talk. Women should wear a bra or support. Stop if you feel any pain.

The purpose is to raise energy, release tension and to break up habitual physical and emotional holding patterns.

relationship with yourself; you become 'full of self'. This change also, inevitably, involves a new relationship with others – including family, friends and colleagues. You will need to recognize and avoid those people who drain your energy. If you have been an 'overcarer', you may find that some members of your family or community resent the change that they see in you. However, on the positive side, the person who is 'full of self' is able to give less conditionally to those around him or her, and indeed can love more fully. This makes sense because, of course, you cannot give from the empty space that is a place of abandonment – the place inhabited by the person of low self-worth. In other words, sometimes it becomes apparent that

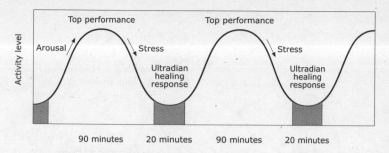

Fig. 8: Graph showing ultradian rhythm

what looked, in the past, like giving, may actually have been taking at the energetic or emotional level.

The Ebb and Flow of Energy

As you become aware of the energy state of body, mind and spirit in different situations, it is important also to be aware of the natural flow of energy at different times of day. These natural activity–rest cycles, called 'ultradian rhythms',[12] occur once every 110 minutes, and are represented in Figure 8 as periods where energy rises to a peak and then wanes, with the need for recovery. Balancing rest and activity, and shifting from doing to being, which many people do naturally in daydreaming, are important in fostering the body's capacity for self-regulation. It can be useful to include in the rest period your meditation or visualization, or a shift to creative activity such as music or dance to restore vitality and energy.

Working with Mind, Body and Spirit

In ancient Greece, when the most revered members of society became ill they were sent – usually for a period of 40 days – to a healing temple, where initially the aim was to avoid all the elements in the business of life which were associated with the

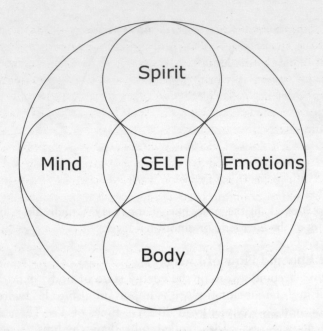

Fig. 9: Mind, body, spirit: the interconnections of the whole person

onset of illness. Body therapies such as massage, hot bathing, herbal oils and sleep, often accompanied by music, were used in the first stages of restoration. After this, when mind and spirit had become stronger, it was possible to look at what might have contributed to the illness. Energy levels would have risen, and then dialogue encouraged individuals to concentrate on and enhance the areas in their lives about which they were really passionate and excited. As the mind and spirit became progressively stronger, the body followed closely behind. (It is one of the ironies of modern Western culture that in the biomedical model we seek ever more sophisticated and expensive drug-based treatments, when in ancient Greece it was the well-to-do members of the society who were restored to wellness in the healing retreat temples while the common populace received medicines!)

At the Centre, in helping you to restore your health, we aim to create an awareness of those things that the mind, body and spirit require to maintain your inner state in balance. When the immune system is working well, it protects us; our natural immune defence cells (T-cells) destroy cancer cells. Recent conventional medical research[13] has shown that when the body's natural T-cell defence system is working well, the cancer responds. We know, too, that the mind–body connection has an influence on these T-cell defence systems. Our need is to understand and foster those factors in our lives that will protect us, restore and/or maintain our well-being, and keep our bodies in anabolic balance. Thus we need to look in detail at the interconnection of mind, body and spirit. These three aspects of us are interdependent. Problems that affect any one of them will also affect the others; and, by the same token, anything that helps any one of them will also assist the others.

Hope and the Will to Live

Spirit or purpose in being determines our will to live.[14] Hope is essential; all those involved in medical practice know that if an individual's spirit has been broken and the will to live has gone, there is no medicine, orthodox or complementary, that will get them well again. So, the role of negative emotions and the ability to recognize how they affect us are crucial in integrative medicine.

The adage 'what the mind represses the body expresses' is borne out in the analysis of case histories. Ian Gawler, in his book *You Can Conquer Cancer*,[15] describes common factors in personality that are recognized by his patients. The pattern that becomes apparent again and again is one in which a tendency to shut down feelings in childhood – maybe because of a discouraging or unappreciative environment – becomes habitual. The adult then develops a tendency to passively serve the needs of others, to be what others seem to want, and a need to be liked. People who take this path become reliant on things outside themselves for a sense of self-worth. Internal resources become correspondingly less robust and diminish over time. When an individual becomes over-reliant on external support, for example from work or a partner, and that is then removed – by, say, redundancy or death – little meaning remains in life. Feelings of hopelessness develop and it becomes impossible to see a viable future. Hopelessness can develop also from a feeling of being trapped, unable to take control of one's circumstances or bring about change.

Many who find themselves in such situations, having spent so long putting other people's needs before their own, preserve a cheery, helpful front despite the encroaching feelings of hopelessness; but inside there is a sense of being shattered. Inwardly, the body can mirror the sense of hopelessness. It is as if the body itself gives up too. It may ultimately lose the will to live and the ability to defend itself as the immune system becomes weakened. We will see in the next section how the young science of psychoneuroimmunology has shown us the mechanisms through which this can happen – and can be prevented or reversed.

'Your Mind is in Every Cell of Your Body': Advances through Psychoneuroimmunology

The term 'psychoneuroimmunology', or PNI, refers to the science that underpins the Bristol Approach. This science was in its infancy when the Centre developed its intuitive approaches to healing; now, in the light of recent advances in PNI, those approaches have been confirmed as valid by scientific research.

Previously the mind – incorporating thoughts, feelings, emotions – was thought to be a separate entity from the body. Then, in the mid-1980s, scientists such as Candace Pert[16] made us aware of the subtle continuous interconnection between mind and body through neurotransmitters called neuropeptides.

These are vast numbers of chemical messengers – specific ones for each emotion – that are in intimate communication with every cell of your body. Pert was the first to discover a receptor or 'switch' in the brain for an opiate-like substance named endorphin. Now over 200 'messenger chemicals' have been discovered. When they interact with the receptors they affect the cells' functioning, either by activating the cells or by slowing down or deactivating them. *So the most immediate way you can influence your immune system is by activating the positive emotions*, prompting the endorphin response that moves throughout the system to influence each cell.

What follows from these discoveries is the profound realization that the intelligence and memory of the human being are not confined to the brain. We can move our body state from defeat or despair to hope and action. Our tissues themselves are intelligent, and even the immune system has the capacity for memory. Robert Adler, in laboratory experiments with rats, found that rats given saccharine combined with an immuno-suppressant drug suffered severe depression in immune function when they were later fed saccharine alone. This demonstrated that the saccharine taste alone triggered the memory of the immune response previously experienced when the rats were fed saccharine. The body had remembered. Conversely, work by Heart Math has shown how positive emotions brought about through awakening heartfelt love and appreciation for the self and others produce increases in well-being, reduce stress and foster the anabolic metabolism.

Cortisol and Depression

The combination of overload accompanied by a sense of defeat or despair[17] – the symptoms typical of depression – causes a rise in the level of a hormone called cortisol. A study carried out by Watson and colleagues[18] among women just six weeks after a diagnosis of breast cancer, with equal disease status when tested, found that those women with a positive depression score

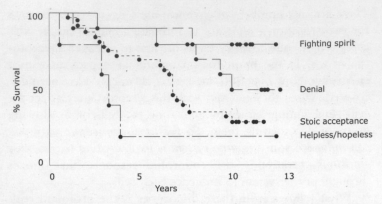

Fig. 10: Comparison of survival rates of women with breast cancer who have different coping styles

survived only half as long as those who were not depressed. This was a study of primary cancer, but Spiegel and colleagues and Sephton and colleagues have found that a raised cortisol level accompanying the diagnosis of secondary cancer also has a similarly adverse effect on outcomes.

Emotions and Survival

The pioneering work of Stephen Greer and colleagues in the 1970s[19] showed how emotional responses to cancer such as helplessness, hopelessness or stoic acceptance reduce survival time (Figure 10). He also found that fighting spirit or positive avoidance (denial) was a helpful strategy. The more recent study by Watson and colleagues confirmed the significantly increased risk of relapse or death in women scoring high on helplessness/hopelessness. Between the time of Greer's study and today, most people have come to know that a fighting spirit or positive attitude is important. However, being pressed to have such an attitude without knowing and feeling what this means, or how to attain it, can simply be another pressure, an extra stress.

Your plan and strategy, and the style that you evolve to live your life in its most effective way, will be helped by the way in which you respond to the challenge. We at the Bristol Cancer Help Centre have the experience, the creative teamwork and support network to help and support you in this process. As science confirms the intuitive knowledge that the Centre has developed over the past 23 years, it becomes ever clearer why it is important to develop the techniques that enable us to maintain a flexible but positive state of mind, and to foster a sense of self-care and love.

Recovery: Discovering What Brings You Alive

Ian Gawler describes his own remarkable recovery from widespread disseminated cancer through intense meditation and reduction of stress; he also describes its recurrence when he became too busy again, and his use of meditation and stress management to overcome it once more. These remain the core therapies in his Australian Yarra Valley retreat centre, as well as in the recovery programmes described in this book.

An essential part of your recovery plan, then, will be to look at your underlying beliefs and attitudes, and consider how these may have led to compulsive patterns of thinking and behaviour which, perhaps without your having fully realized it, have taken a central position in your life. Thus you will be able to work towards a new coping style to confront the threat from your illness.

> I realized that I really had to make life changes. I had always been a yes person; people would phone me up all hours of the day and night and 'Yes, Jenny would do it', even if nobody else would. I couldn't say no to people. Afterwards I would put the phone down and wish I had thought about it. I realized that I had never put myself first – I was always worrying about other people.
>
> *Jenny Jackson, living with liver cancer, first diagnosed in 1987*

The best way to make the mind–body connection work to your benefit is to discover what really brings you alive. Laurence LeShan, in his book *You Can Fight for Your Life*,[20] describes remarkable recoveries when each person rediscovers and starts to 'sing his or her own song'. Creative therapies such as art, music and dance may assist greatly with this process.

The Use of Therapies in Mind–Body Interaction

When we use the power of our mind in visualization, the communication between mind and body affects the state of our immune system. Professor Leslie Walker and colleagues[21] evaluated the effects of relaxation training and guided imagery on quality of life and response to primary chemotherapy in women with locally advanced breast cancer. Women received six cycles of chemotherapy, surgery, hormone therapy and radiotherapy. In addition they were allocated randomly to one of two groups: one that received a high level of support in the form of access to a cancer nurse and counselling, and one that received identical support plus relaxation and guided imagery. It was found that women in the latter group, using relaxation and guided imagery, had significantly improved mood, and responded better to chemotherapy. The effect on immune function was to increase the number and proportion of T-cells, the 'killer cells' of the immune system that attack the cancer. The natural activity of these killer cells was found to be significantly higher in those women who rated the quality of imagery highly.

There is also evidence that meeting our need to touch and talk, to reveal our inner self to others, is important. The research of Spiegel[22] showed that 'supportive expressive work' in small groups for those with secondary cancer significantly increases survival. Fawzy-Fawzy confirms these results;[23] in his study, a weekly 90-minute session of similar work was accompanied by a significant improvement in survival among individuals with malignant melanoma. We know, too, that keeping a journal, in which negative thoughts are disclosed, is effective

Exercises in mind–body interaction
One simple exercise described by the American physician
Naras Bhat in his book *How to Reverse and Prevent Heart
Disease and Cancer* is as follows:[24]

- Focus awareness in the area of your anatomical heart.
- Ask yourself: Can I experience caring love?
- Bring back a memory of a place where you have felt loved
  and appreciated.
- Stay anchored to your heart and observe your breathing
  and how it centres in your belly.

It may be helpful to see how a mind–body exercise using software and a computer changes our internal states: Heart Math
and Better Physiology[25] have developed appropriate software
designed for educational use and Heart Math has a series of
interactive games that show your mind–body connection
working.

at elevating mood and preventing depression, while art therapy has been shown to be particularly effective at releasing sup-
pressed emotion and freeing people from a negative self-image.

'Hexing' and the Benefits of Hypnosis
On the positive side, then, the evidence is clear and com-
pelling. Similar evidence is available to show how the
mind–body connection can work negatively when inappropri-
ate approaches are taken, for example in communicating a
diagnosis of cancer. 'Hexing' is a term used to refer to the
instilling of belief in the giver of bad news. Often – in good
faith – professionals or friends offer the bad news of a cancer
diagnosis to a person in a state of high stress and consequent
emotional arousal. For some people this news, given when
they are vulnerable, can go deep within the subconscious and
be acted out in confirming the 'prophecy'. Many people are
sent into a state of 'hypnosis' by the shock of the diagnosis

and the memory of the implied or perceived poor outcome is then ingrained. If this may have occurred in your experience, then you may well benefit from medical hypnosis, where the internal state is altered to one of calm, and positive thoughts replace the negative.

I have referred earlier in this chapter to the work of Alastair Cunningham. He has shown that in secondary cancer it is necessary to work particularly hard to reverse previous patterning.

Putting all these elements together, it becomes apparent how great the benefits can be of a programme such as that recommended by Spiegel, where as well as support and mind–body techniques such as relaxation, the teaching of self-hypnosis and bodywork, there is a safe space to share experiences, both negative and positive.

Awareness of Our Own Mortality – the 'Yielding' Style

We are all mortal, and a diagnosis of cancer brings us face to face with this reality. Research by Cunningham shows that,[26] far from it being morbid to contemplate our own end, it is healthy to face it and to prepare for what is, after all, ultimately inevitable for everyone. So, in this 'yielding' approach we allow ourselves to face the possibility of dying: to make our preparations, to make peace with others, and ourselves, and to let those whom we love know that we love and care for them. Thus we create the possibility of letting go with love, and also of letting our loved ones know that we wish to live fully and joyfully for whatever time remains to us, however long or short it may be.

Putting it All Together

The cancer diagnosis brings with it a strong threat to our very being. The threat brings with it the possibility of dying, and a remembrance that we all, in the end, die. Our ability to cope and deal with the threat is likely to be helped considerably by awareness of the interacting influences that go to make up our own unique way of dealing with the threat brought about by the cancer diagnosis. We can then choose interventions, within a framework of support.

Your plan will acknowledge that you have become the greatest expert when it comes to your needs. The aim of the second part of this book is to help you reflect on your current situation and to develop the right strategy. As we come to understand the way mind and body communicate, so we come to understand how we can develop a new and healing relationship with our body, *of which the cancer is only a part.*

We can harness resources from inside us, and from the outer world, through our support networks. We can work with conventional treatment in an integrative partnership, retaining a sense of control. The combination of approaches, following the whole-person model, is likely to prove more effective than pursuing one on its own in generating increased well-being, quality of life and – as the growing body of evidence suggests – survival.

3
Complementary Therapies and Self-help Techniques in Holistic Cancer Care

This chapter aims to describe the types of therapies used at Bristol and elsewhere in holistic care of people with cancer. This will give you an idea of the variety of therapies and techniques available to you, and enable you to understand them more fully so that you can design an appropriate package of care for yourself.

The Doctors at the Bristol Cancer Help Centre

The doctors at the Centre provide a bridge between the worlds of mainstream and complementary medicine, supporting you in the process of taking charge of your situation, and working step by step towards the recovery of health. They will help in the initial evaluation of the state of your mind, body and spirit, as well as in the process of sorting out what your therapeutic and self-help plan should be according to your needs at the time of consultation. This will also involve helping you to choose the right complementary medicines should they be appropriate.

These doctors can also help you to take time to understand your illness and its treatment, and to assess the medical options you are being given, counselling you through the process of making truly informed decisions about the treatments you are being offered. Advice on the tailoring of nutritional approaches to your specific medical conditions and fine-tuning your nutritional supplementation regime of vitamins, minerals and other natural medicines is usually also included, as are suggestions for symptom control by complementary means.

The Nurses at the Bristol Cancer Help Centre

The nurses at the Centre provide care, advice and support to those attending the courses and help to control symptoms with natural medicines, massage and self-help techniques. As the nurses have a background of working with and supporting cancer patients in both orthodox and complementary settings, they are in the unique position of being able to fully integrate their conventional medical knowledge and experience with the holistic approach offered at the Centre. This means that patients can feel fully supported in any choice they make about conventional and/or complementary treatment.

The nurses will often be able to help patients to control symptoms through the use of visualization, massage, relaxation and breathing techniques, and comforting support. Further improvement may be gained through the use of natural remedies drawn from the spectrum of herbal medicine, homoeopathy and Bach Flower Remedies.

Counselling

When confronted by serious illness it is important to be able to talk about those things that are very important to us, our lives and those we are close to. Thoughts and questions will naturally arise relating to the illness, its treatment, the effects of both illness and treatment on everyday life and relationships, the changes that will need to be absorbed and possible short- and long-term outcomes. The changes and challenges that a life-threatening illness forces upon us can initially summon up thoughts and emotions that may be very new to us; these emotions can be unpredictable, and not the least of them is the fear of death and of an uncertain future.

Support through talking is crucial. It can help us become aware of what we need to do, initially in learning to sort out what our questions might be and how we might go about getting the answers. Talking about our situation can also help us to unravel our thinking and settle our minds, while enabling us to explore our feelings and emotions and those aspects of ourselves that we may call spirit or soul, or our deeper self. Counselling is a method through which we can begin this process, giving us an opportunity to find understanding and bring greater clarity to our unique situation, in order to re-establish our sense of control of our life and world.

Counselling within a holistic, mind–body–spirit model is considered a central component of the healing process. During a counselling session the emphasis is on seeking to explore gently and safely, principally through conversation, those things that are important and relevant to the effects and changes that the cancer has brought about in everyday life and significant relationships.

There are many counselling styles and models to chose from. The holistic model established at the Bristol Cancer Help Centre, used in both one-to-one counselling and group therapy, is termed 'transpersonal'. Transpersonal counselling[27] seeks to help the individual to explore his or her needs from a whole-person perspective. Serious illness challenges all parts of our being: our physical body, our thoughts, our feelings, our emotions, our spirit, our significant relationships and the environments in which we live. Initially, the need is to cope with the crisis of diagnosis and the grief surrounding the loss of the known, and to explore the potential adjustments involved in facing a new reality. As those adjustments take place, so counselling can become a more expansive and co-creative experience.

A transpersonal counselling approach is a creative one. In addition to talking, there is opportunity to access different aspects of ourselves which may be found through the use of guided imagery, visualizations, working with images and symbols which can arise within our dreams and daydreams, artwork, writing and keeping a personal journal, and learning relaxation. These approaches are both enlightening and supportive, and encourage us to use all of ourselves when dealing with crisis, adjusting to change. They allow us to learn to be in touch with ourselves at all levels of our being and life.

Through counselling of this kind, we can learn especially to listen to our own inner voices and the guidance and intuition we can offer ourselves. Our inner wisdom is often very underused in our normal busy way of being; very often we don't know how far we can grow and cope until we are faced with a serious challenge that invites us to call on our own inner resources while receiving help from a trained and experienced counsellor alongside other supporters. Transpersonal counselling always seeks to aid and assist without creating dependency on the counsellor. In crisis situations it is especially helpful to be able to access these parts of ourselves so that we can make the decisions that are truly congruent with our innermost sense of what is right for us and what will help us begin to be well again.

Most people think that counselling is about the relief of emotional distress only, but transpersonal counselling is very much about helping us to see again what aspects of ourselves are right and strong, as well as helping us to re-identify with our true nature and more authentic sense of self.

The counsellor can act as a mirror, helping us to see what we know to be true about ourselves, particularly seeing the patterns or ties or counterproductive situations from which we need to be released, so that our life and energies will start to flow freely again.

Through this type of counselling, what we know and feel can be revealed, and connections made, very quickly. We can be helped to identify what our soul and spirit are yearning for – which may even be to let go and die. Although on the surface we may seem to be actively fighting illness, at a deeper level we may have made quite a different choice; if so, by connecting to our deeper reality through counselling, great truth and peace can be established.

Conversely, we may be yearning quite literally to come back to life, and rediscover our passion and potential as we take new directions, or fulfil our most important needs and ambitions. For those afraid of death and dying, being able to confront those fears (which may have been affecting their life for many years) often liberates an enormous new lease of life as the fear dissipates.

Counselling also provides an environment in which we can look at our relationships. We can find out whether we have become stuck, losing tremendous amounts of energy by repeating the same unsatisfactory relationship patterns over and over again. We can also look at extended features of our personality, known as 'sub-personalities', of which there may be many. Often there is a bossy, dominant or highly critical sub-personality which is overshadowing a gentler, more creative aspect of ourselves; or an over-serious, over-responsible part that is overshadowing a playful, creative or humorous aspect of ourselves. As our awareness is increased, we learn how to soften, reduce or strengthen the qualities and characteristics of these parts of our personality, so that we can then learn to live more wholesome lives, more in touch with who we really are. This can help us to find and liberate our greater potential for health and well-being, while bringing our life back into balance.

I have been a very rational and organized person all of my life. I was loath to accept anything that was not provable and logical. I would never have considered asking for help, I just preferred to sort myself out, either by settling it through reasoning it out or just ignore the problem. When I became ill I was greatly suspicious of counselling. I could not understand how talking about my situation was going to change it, that was the job of the treatment only. So I entered the counselling with great hesitation and not sure if I wanted to cooperate. But I was surprised to find that I found it very helpful. I imagined that I would have to 'bare my soul' and lose control, but that was not what happened. I felt comfortable to be able to gradually talk about myself, at my pace. The counsellor seemed to know how to give me their attention without dictating how things should go. I needed some help to direct my thoughts and feelings and found this was structured in to the counselling so well.

At first I was unsure how to express myself, but soon I found that I was able to express myself in my own way and to come to some resolution over my situation. I continued to see a counsellor and am so much enjoying the whole process. It has helped me to talk to my wife and to understand her better and to be able to show my emotions more and to take for myself. I find talking, coupled with keeping a daily journal of my experiences and my reactions to them, plus the visualizations and relaxations I do with the help of the counsellor and on my own are helping me to balance my life and face things in a more balanced way. My cancer has not gone away completely but I am learning to live with it and to know myself for the first time in my life.

Tom, 55-year-old, self-employed, living with cancer of the liver, first diagnosed in 1999

Group Therapy

Another helpful form of counselling is the 'solution-focused approach'. This was developed in America in the 1980s on the basis of two simple ideas. First, the therapist helps individuals to explore how they are handling their problems and to reflect back to a time when they were confronting these problems effectively; the aim is thus to help them to discover what abilities they already have that may contribute to their ability to cope with present challenges. Second, the therapist helps the person to explore what life might be like for them if these problems were solved – on the understanding that, although it may not be possible to change the actual situation facing them (such as a diagnosis of cancer), it may be possible to change their attitude towards it. By focusing on solutions in this way, the aim is to give both therapist and client a picture of the most effective way forward.

Getting to know and understand ourselves better can also take place within a context of mutual support among people in similar situations to our own. It can be extremely helpful to meet and talk with people who have the same problems or needs as ourselves. The sense of identification, support and solidarity that can be engendered within a group of people sharing their individual experiences can be an enormously helpful process. Both the individual and the group as a whole can be compassionately engaged with and focused on the things that are important for understanding and can assist in the short- and long-term healing process. This form of counselling or therapy, often called 'group therapy', provides many people with an enormous sense of relief from the isolation and alienation that they feel, especially when they have a serious illness.

Although the aim of group therapy is not to expose feelings, it can, perhaps surprisingly, be easier to let go and express your emotions with the support of the group than it is with friends or family, or even in a one-to-one session with a therapist or counsellor. It can also be very constructive to work together to identify needs and common underlying beliefs and patterns which may be obstructing progress towards self-acceptance and well-being. With the mutual support and encouragement provided by members of the group, individuals can often feel bold enough to express creative ideas about new values and priorities, as well as learning self-help techniques together.

This type of group therapy is facilitated by an experienced counsellor or psychotherapist. Other groups aimed at accessing mutual support are run on a more social basis, but are nevertheless of great value, particularly for continuous long-term support. These groups often share resources, can be helpful over practical problems (they are often good sources of information at the local level), can be a link to other organizations, and frequently offer support for family and other significant members within members' personal networks.

I am not used to talking about myself in a group of people. As a teacher I was the one in control. When I sat for the first time in the group I felt self-conscious and wondered what other people were thinking. Some were talking and expressing themselves so well, I was not sure if I wanted to say how I was feeling. But as I listened, I found that others were almost speaking out loud what I was feeling. I found this so reassuring, that I was not on my own in the way some of my thoughts and feelings had been since my diagnosis and treatment. I could not at home speak about my fear or grief; everyone knew me as a positive, get-up-and-go person, and so I had had to keep up that front, when actually I didn't feel positive at all. I needed to stop and be allowed to say what I was really feeling.

I did finally collect my courage and I spoke out. I found that what I said was received with respect and support. I felt that the group of people was so mixed – ages, backgrounds, types of cancer – but somehow within the differences there was a bond. It wasn't all gloom and doom: we laughed, we pulled

each other's legs and we cried, and the sense of companionship was so very healing for me.
Jenny, 35-year-old school teacher, living with breast cancer, first diagnosed in 2000

Creative Therapies

The creative therapies used at the Bristol Cancer Help Centre are art and music. These can be extremely freeing, allowing people to express what they may find difficult to put into words. They require no previous skill or expertise, and can often be linked very successfully with group therapeutic work, deepening the experience and giving an outlet for insights that arise through visualization processes or individual psychotherapeutic work.

Creative therapies can also rejuvenate the more playful, joyful, creative aspects of our natures, enabling us to capture again the feelings of energy and fun that we took for granted in youth.

Art Therapy

A diagnosis of cancer, and all the treatments and interventions that may accompany it, can leave people feeling that they have little choice about what is happening in their lives. They may feel that they are no longer able to be creative about how they are living. The Bristol Cancer Help Centre uses art therapy as a way of reconnecting individuals with their own inner resources of creativity. Work done in art therapy can help people discover a sense of control and empowerment in their life; it can also be cathartic, releasing, surprising, spiritual, absorbing, fun, difficult and emotional! This is the wonder of creating art: it can have many different, simultaneous meanings and contain mixtures of feelings that can sometimes be overwhelming.

Many people naturally feel some apprehension about doing

artwork, especially if they have not done any for some time – if ever. But no art skill is needed, and most people find that, once they involve themselves in using paints, clay, paper, glue or whatever they choose, they become absorbed and involved. This is beneficial in its own right, giving the mind a rest from its habitual whirring. It's very different from an art class – all work is accepted as an authentic, meaningful part of the 'artist'.

One participant described her work as 'a journey of hope. I drew a forest in which I was lost, and a mountain of fear. Then came a river of hope, a life and healing. There are new shoots of wisdom growing beside it.' Another person found while using clay that he was modelling his own body: 'I soothed and smoothed it, distancing myself from the pain. By facing how my body feels now I was able to transform it.' Of her painting of a garden viewed through a window, one participant commented: 'I can go into that garden, not stay shut inside. I can walk along that path – the vivid colours are really important. It's joy, peace.'

Art therapy at the Bristol Cancer Help Centre is carried out in small groups run by an art therapist. It is also possible to use art processes in this way while at home or undergoing treatment. Some suggestions for individual work are given in the self-help guide in Part Two of this book (see pp. 147–9); it may also be helpful to consult an art therapist at some point while doing this.

Art therapy is becoming increasingly used by people with cancer, both during and after treatment, in hospitals and other centres across the world. One of many examples is the art therapy done by bone-marrow transplant patients at the Memorial Sloan-Kettering Cancer Center, New York, during their long time in isolation.[28] The art therapists found that the participants used art therapy to 'fulfil a variety of emotional needs: (a) to strengthen positive thoughts, (b) to resolve distressing emotional conflicts, (c) to deepen the awareness of existential and spiritual issues, and (d) to facilitate communication with relative and friends.'

We all have a creative instinct, which may take different forms. Making art is a wonderful way of communicating our inner world, to both ourselves and others. In the words of Jung, 'the happy state is the creative state.'

Music and Music Therapy

Music therapy[29] has always played an integral part in the Bristol Approach. A group session takes place on Wednesday afternoon, almost at the mid-point of the five-day course (see above, pp. 16–18). The Centre has a wide range of tuned and untuned percussion instruments from all corners of the world. These instruments are very accessible, and no previous musical training is needed to take full advantage of the session. Music has a long history of links with healing processes, and we find that making music together helps people to express feelings that may be difficult to put into words. Very often we find that participants in the sessions are able to use what they discover through the music in the rest of the week at the Centre, as the music contributes to the group work.

We have found that music can both reduce physical tensions and increase energy levels. It can relieve anxiety, or help people to express confused and angry feelings. People attending the music therapy sessions often comment how the music lifts them on to another plane, helping to alleviate any pain while the music lasts. The session can also be a lot of fun, as inhibitions are lost and people join in what is very much a social activity.

In addition to the active playing, sessions usually include some time for listening to music in a very relaxed state. The session is led by a state registered music therapist who has an additional training in guided imagery and music. Some suggestions on using listening to music as a self-help technique are given if requested.

Over the last few years we have been carrying out some collaborative research into how both active playing and listening can help people. We have found, for example, that people feel better about themselves after the music sessions. There is less tension after listening and an increase in energy after playing. We have also done some preliminary work exploring how some of these positive psychological shifts link with physiological boosts to the immune system, even after listening for just a short period.

During the five-day course at the Centre, other staff besides the music therapist may use music as a focus for meditation or to help with movement work. Musicians are also invited into the Centre to play after supper, and these evenings of relaxed listening have proved to be a very positive and enjoyable part of the programme.

Spiritual Healing

In an elegant and convincing, albeit small, piece of research published in 1998 by the Royal Society of Medicine, a GP, Dr Michael Dixon, showed unequivocally that patients receiving healing in his practice, and who had not had relief from conventional medicine in over five years of treatment, experienced a reduction of over 50 per cent in their symptoms and distress, and equally significant drops in their usage of medication after only ten healing sessions.[30] A recent systematic review of trials conducted on a variety of forms of distant healing (prayer, therapeutic touch, spiritual healing) demonstrated that 57 per cent of the trials showed a positive effect for a variety of different medical conditions.[31]

Spiritual healing (also called laying on of hands, natural healing, contact healing or therapeutic touch) is the oldest of the healing arts. It is at the heart of many religions and belief systems, founded on the principle that we are One, and that reconnecting to the source heals.

Healing is brought about by priest, healer, being prayed for – or directly, by personal prayer and self-healing exercises.

Healers believe that the universal life force, which unites us as one, often becomes depleted. The healers' skill and experience enables them to tune in, through focus of intention, and bring this loving energy to whomever needs it, to restore balance to body, mind and spirit.

Healing has the remarkable effect of raising energy levels greatly while simultaneously calming and lifting the spirit. While healers themselves have their own specific belief systems, they are discouraged through their code of ethics from sharing these beliefs with their clients, aiming to keep the healing environment as neutral as possible. From the recipient's point of view, then, the healing is entirely non-denominational, beyond any personal religion or belief system, a completely natural, universal connection with the spiritual quality of each person. However, where people do have strong religious beliefs it is possible to find a healer who is of their own spiritual affiliation, and this can provide a very safe and reinforcing environment for the individual's spiritual belief and practice.

I was very wary when I had my first healing experience. I didn't know what to expect. But I went in open-minded, and I was very nicely surprised. It was this feeling of calmness and peacefulness that I felt instantly. I continued having healing over a long period of time, about once a week for two years. It was always this feeling of stillness – it was a very positive experience. It helped me to be empowered really – to continue with the fighting spirit and to get well again.
Jenny Jackson, living with liver cancer, first diagnosed in 1987

The Energy Medicines

Energy medicines can play a crucial role in the rebalancing and recharging of your system. The best-known classical systems are acupuncture, shiatsu and homoeopathy, all of which work to balance and restore the flow of the vital energy in the body.

Acupuncture

Acupuncture originated in China. The acupuncture therapist uses very fine needles that are inserted into the skin at points found along the energy channels within the body. It is used to rebalance the energy flow in the body's meridians (energy channels).

Shiatsu

Shiatsu is a form of acupressure that originated in Japan. It combines healing touch with subtle energy rebalancing.

A fuller description of use of shiatsu at the Centre is given in the section on bodywork at the bottom of this page.

Homoeopathy

The principle of homoeopathy, which has its origins in Europe, is that 'like cures like'. This means that the symptoms that a particular substance produces can be cured by that same substance if it is given in homoeopathically prepared doses. Homoeopathic medicines support the person's underlying constitution, strengthening their 'vital force' and ability to combat disease. They are given in the form of tiny pills, which are prescribed after very detailed and precise consultation with a homoeopath or holistic doctor.

Bodywork

The Role of Bodywork at the Bristol Cancer Help Centre

At the Centre we have long recognized that the caring touch of a holistic bodyworker can act as a powerful catalyst for healing. Massage[32] and shiatsu can help you reconnect with your body and soothe the hurt and isolation arising from the cancer and its treatment. Touch can relieve physical symptoms, help release emotions and rebuild self-esteem.

The massage practitioner will generally work with oil, using gentle stroking, light pressure and stretching to improve your body's circulation, promote deep physical and mental relaxation, and release emotional hurt. We also use specialized techniques for scar tissue and lymphoedema, where appropriate.

The shiatsu practitioner works through your clothing on a mat or futon on the floor. Techniques such as gently applied pressure, holding and stretching are used to encourage your life energy (*chi*) to flow. This process is enhanced through the use of the meridian system to influence the internal organs, encouraging healing and balance. Every treatment is specific to the individual. Gentle touch allows for a depth of stillness to be experienced, where the body's own healing power can be activated.

After a shiatsu treatment it is common to experience a deep feeling of relaxation, although sometimes old feelings/emotions may surface, requiring to be relinquished in order that a deeper healing can take place.

Benefits of Bodywork
Our experience at the Bristol Cancer Help Centre shows us that regular bodywork sessions can lead to improved confidence, ease with emotional expression and a renewed sense of hope. There is also a growing body of research evidence which supports the value of massage. Studies show that having a massage can help you by:

- relaxing stiff muscles,[33] reducing blood pressure, nausea, fatigue, insomnia, oedema and pain;
- relieving constipation,[34] improving blood and lymph circulation, stimulating the immune system, reducing shock and headaches and improving appetite;

- reducing shock, fear, tension, stress and anxiety;[35]
- releasing areas of blocked energy,[36] revitalizing and balancing;
- increasing feelings of calmness,[37] relaxation, physical (non-sexual) pleasure, improving body image, self-awareness and self-esteem;
- increasing the number of natural killer (NK) cells in the immune system[38] and reducing stress hormones;
- reducing anxiety, depression and pain;[39]
- for people undergoing chemotherapy,[40] reducing nausea and vomiting more effectively and cheaply then medication.

Concerns about Bodywork

You may have heard that massage might spread cancer around the body through the lymphatic vessels. We know of no scientific evidence to support this assertion. Indeed, many oncology specialists these days are supportive of touch for their patients; it is mostly within the bodywork community that the fear is perpetuated.

The view that massage is entirely ruled out for people with cancer may have arisen when massage was primarily associated with brisk, forceful, deep work of the kind a football team's physiotherapist might do! This would certainly not be appropriate for someone whose body was being challenged by cancer; but there are now many other gentle, non-invasive approaches to massage which are particularly appropriate.

Choosing a Bodywork Therapist

Your bodyworker can become a valued companion on your journey with cancer (the word 'therapy' comes from the Greek *therapoa*, meaning to accompany). So, when choosing a therapist outside Bristol, make sure you feel comfortable with the individual concerned. Ask how much experience this person has. It is important that the therapist is able be flexible, adapting to each individual's situation as it evolves. Generally, at Bristol we recommend that bodywork practitioners should have at least two years' post-qualification experience.

Also, ask what training the bodyworker has had. A shiatsu practitioner should be a member of the professional register of the Shiatsu Society (MRSS). The world of massage is diverse, so ask practitioners if they adopt a holistic approach to their work and what they understand by that. The holistic practitioner does massage 'with' clients, not 'to' them. At Bristol we insist on the highest standard of training, such as that set by the Massage Training Institute (MTI).

Furthermore, a good bodywork therapist needs sufficient life experience and interpersonal skills to support you during the process of your sessions together. It is essential that body-workers in the field of cancer care should be receiving continuing supervision and also receive regular bodywork themselves.

The Link between Nutrition and Cancer

When the Bristol Cancer Help Centre opened in 1980, the idea that cancer and nutrition were linked was considered irrational, and the giving of vitamin and mineral supplements was thought by orthodox doctors to be a waste of time and money. Now, mainstream cancer authorities assert that the poor nutrition associated with Western dietary habits causes 30–40 per cent of cancer mortality in the West.[41] This makes it the highest cause of all (the second highest, at 30 per cent, is smoking). In 1994 Drs Key and Thorogood reported that,[42] having followed 11,000 vegetarians for 17 years they had observed a 25 per cent lower incidence of death from heart disease, 32 per cent lower death rate from strokes, and 40–50 per cent lower death rate from cancer than in their meat-eating (but otherwise matched) counterparts.

It would appear that the evidence is strong that vegetables

and fruit are almost invariably protective against most major cancers, and high consumption of meat – especially red and processed meat – is linked to the risk of bowel, breast, prostate and pancreatic cancer. Obesity and alcohol consumption[43] are also associated with increased risk. There have also been some extremely interesting investigations into the link between dairy produce and breast cancer.[44] It is far more complex to study the effect of nutrition on a tumour once cancer has developed. It would seem sensible, however, to presume that nutritional factors that have been shown to be effective to prevent cancer developing might be significant in promoting health and regeneration for people who have developed cancer.

With regard to vitamin and mineral supplementation, there have been some 10,000 scientific studies looking at the effects of, particularly, the antioxidants C, E, bcta-carotene, selenium and zinc on prevention and reversal of cancer. The vast majority of these show encouraging results, the only concern being that it is inadvisable to take synthetic beta-carotene supplements if you are a smoker as it appears to make things worse rather than better. (Bristol therefore recommends supplements made from naturally occurring beta-carotene.) Most encouraging is an American study conducted in China,[45] which showed that taking the vitamins and minerals A, C, E and selenium reduced the overall death rate from cancer by 13 per cent, and by 20 per cent in their two most common cancers (of the stomach and oesophagus).

The most recent discoveries in the field are showing that it is not just the vitamins and minerals in plant foods that protect us from cancer but also several large families of plant chemicals that are known collectively as phytochemicals. There are many different mechanisms of action involved in this protective effect, but some of these chemicals can actually stabilize and repair DNA and RNA in cell nuclei, preventing and reversing the genetic changes that allow cell lines to become cancerous. This is a staggering discovery: it means that we have to change our image of vegetables as simply being good for our hair and skin to being the absolutely core, vital element in protecting and repairing our cells from dangerous genetic mutation. This is no doubt why there have been highly unexpected recoveries in people who put themselves on to rigorous fruit and vegetable fasts and juicing regimes, such as the Gerson diet.

However, to date, we cannot predict which cancers and which individuals will respond to such diets, and further work needs to be done to continue to identify the most potent plant chemicals and their mechanisms of action for cellular repair and protection. The phytochemicals currently under investigation are indole-glycosinates found in green leafy vegetables and broccoli; phyto-oestrogens found in soya products; phytates, lignans, protease inhibitors, isoflavonoids and isoflavones, which are present in many plant foods and are thought to be inhibitors of oncogenes (the genes that make you predisposed to cancer). Limonene (contained in lemons) and lycopene (in tomatoes) are also anti-cancer phytochemicals, and substances found in shiitake mushrooms and the seaweeds kombu and kelp interfere with the initiation and promotion of cancer cells.

Other plant-chemical families under study are plant phenols, aromatic isothyocyanates, methylated flavones, coumarines and plant sterols, as well as the naturally occurring plant selenium salts, the vitamin C family, with all the accompanying bioflavonoids and cofactors (now thought to be as important as the vitamin itself), and the tocopherols, retinols and carotenes.

In the meantime, it is absolutely clear that high levels of plant material in the diet are quite essential for our health if we are trying to fight or prevent cancer. Carcinogenic contaminants exist in the general environment, and may also be present in the home or workplace; they may be created through cooking, food preparation and storage processes, and can gain access to the body via food, air or water. They can also be ingested with tobacco smoke, alcohol and drugs, as well as via radiation and cellular toxins that are accumulated during medical procedures and treatments. Plant phytochemicals materials serve both to protect our cells and to render innocuous any potentially carcinogenic substances ingested into the body.

Nutritional Therapy

There are many nutritional therapeutic approaches to illness, where food itself is used as the medicine. The best-known of these are naturopathy, macrobiotics, fasting, juice diets and, in the cancer world, the Gerson diet. The challenge with such diets is that although there have been some thought-provoking successes, minimal clinical results exist to strongly support their use. This is not to say that they do not work; just that there has not been a lot of research into these therapies. Some extremely interesting research, however, has been conducted recently exploring the use of an alternative diet for people with inoperable pancreatic cancer that includes large doses of proteolytic enzymes, along with diet, nutritional supplements and 'detoxification' procedures.[46] The results appear promising, with people outliving their prognosis. It is clear that we need far more of this type and calibre of research exploring the value of these alternative diets.

At Bristol, if people express a wish to follow such diets, we refer them to people who are able to assist them; they are counselled, however, that such diets are rigorous and demand a great deal of application.

The Nutritional Policy of the Bristol Cancer Help Centre

Many people prefer to adopt a more long-term healthy eating approach designed to promote rehabilitation and regeneration, and to improve health and nutritional status. This is now the policy of the Bristol Centre. The healthy eating approach at Bristol stresses the importance of making sure you eat vegetables and fruit, widely varied and preferably organic, with every meal. It is also important to eat food that is not processed and does not contain food additives, and to take, where possible, the wholefood or 'brown' option (brown rice, wholegrain bread, wholemeal flour, and so on). At the same time, efforts must be made to minimize the animal produce consumed in the diet, particularly the amount of animal fat. Sugar and salt intake should also be reduced, as should the consumption of stimulants such as coffee, tea and alcohol. (For more detail on the Centre's nutritional policy, see Appendix 1.)

> When I came on the course at Bristol I realized very quickly how important the diet was. It was surprisingly easy for me to make the change to being a vegan. It also felt like a very positive thing to do. I went home and gave up certain foods, which weren't doing me any good, made the changes, and very quickly afterwards I started feeling a lot better – mentally, because it was good actually doing something constructive, and physically, because my energy got better. So overall it was a very profound thing for me to do.
> *Jenny Jackson, living with liver cancer, first diagnosed in 1987*

The problem in the West is that we are simultaneously overfed and undernourished: this is because we eat very high-calorie foods, full of fat and sugar, but lacking sufficient vitamins, minerals and the vital plant chemicals that we need to stay healthy and protected from heart disease and cancer.

One of the keys to changing diet successfully is to add the extra fruit, vegetables and juices before taking other things away, so that the changeover is gradual and there is no feeling of deprivation. When people first start to eat well, they may experience some weight loss, but this should stabilize as the healthy diet becomes established. The important thing here is not to forget to eat enough carbohydrates and vegetable oils (in the form of pasta, grains and bread, olive and linseed oils), especially if weight loss is already a problem. Some people can become so focused on the raw vegetable and juice components of their new diet that they forget to eat enough 'energy foods' that provide the necessary calories.

If possible, start growing your own food. Even if you do not have a vegetable garden, it is worth growing herbs or sprouts in the kitchen or on the windowsill, or even intermingling vegetables with flowers in hanging baskets and flowerbeds.

If you are worried at all about changes in your body as a result of changing your diet, you should immediately consult a holistic doctor or nutritionist.

Recommended Supplements

The Bristol Cancer Help Centre recommends the antioxidant vitamins and minerals A, C and E, zinc and selenium, and vitamin B complex. Vitamin A is given as its safe precursor, beta-carotene, in its natural form. This regime is often supplemented with co-enzyme Q10 to help energize the intracellular respiratory/energy-producing mechanisms. Dosage instructions are given in the introductory pack that you can obtain at the Centre, either in the shop or by mail order. Dosages are not included in this book as we change our recommendations from time to time in the light of new research.

Herbal Medicine

Help can be gained from herbal medicine, either European or Oriental. Here traditional remedies are chosen for their role in aiding specific conditions and symptoms. They can be particularly effective in cleansing the body and strengthening the tissues, and in soothing inflammation.

Self-help Techniques

Exercise

Once you are strong enough you may wish to replace or augment bodywork and energy medicines with Eastern exercise practices, which keep the energy flow moving and balanced. Those used as part of the Bristol Approach are the systems of tai chi, chi gong and yoga – all wonderfully integrated holistic practices that stimulate the body and rebalance the system, keep the *chi* flowing in the body and clear the mind, engendering an extremely peaceful state of being.

Within yoga there is a sub-speciality called 'pranayama', which is very specialized breathwork. This can be enormously helpful for people with breathing problems, and for anyone who needs to calm their nervous system and to re-energize themselves. We also encourage swimming and walking in order to develop strength and stamina.

Mind–Body Techniques

The other extremely important self-help techniques are the mind–body techniques of relaxation, meditation and visualization. Overall, these techniques have the effect of lessening the grip of fear in our bodies and minds, so that the spirit lifts and the body is able to relax and heal.

There is a fascinating body of research evidence to support the use of these therapies. Studies have shown a positive effect for the control of physical symptoms,[47] for example, chemotherapy-induced nausea; also for assisting emotional distress and promoting adjustment. There have also been surprising results showing a survival advantage for people with lymphoma who use such techniques.[48]

There can be a tendency for these specialities to blur into one, but in reality they are very different and should be treated as such, because they all have specific and extremely important therapeutic values.

Relaxation Relaxation can be said to help us to achieve inner balance,[49] free from striving and distraction, so that we can fully experience and appreciate the very moment that we are in.

The principle of relaxation is that if you can learn to recognize the changing states in your body, particularly the building up of tension, strain, stress or pain, you can respond more quickly to relieve it. So often we do not feel tension until it has become established, and it then becomes difficult to find relief from it. It is important, therefore, to take time to tune in to your body.

Holistic approaches recognize the connectedness and the communication that exist between the body and the mind. So, while relaxation is one way of responding principally to the immediate needs of the body, helping to reduce physical tension and stress, there is a positive consequential effect of releasing similar tensions from within the whole person: mind, emotions, thought processes and spirit too. Relaxation techniques assist the body to withdraw from activity, resulting in a calming effect which leads to the rebalancing of the whole self. This is known as the 'relaxation response'.

Relaxation is a skill, and needs practice for the effects of the relaxation response to have maximum benefit over time. There are many ways to achieve this physical response. One simple method is known as 'progressive muscular relaxation'. This approach is very easy to learn and to do. It involves releasing tension in one group of muscles at a time, until the body becomes softer and there is a often a physical sense of heaviness in the limbs and throughout the body as a whole. As you make your way through this simple technique you will notice that you will automatically move into an unfocused, pleasant state of mind. With each sequential step you will be entering the relaxation response, leading to additional feelings of warmth and comfort, and possibly going into a light state of sleep. Indeed, some people often use this particular relaxation technique to help them to go to sleep. It is certainly a common experience for many people to fall asleep following or even during the relaxation process. In many instances sleep is much needed, and its quality is often improved by the introduction of a relaxation programme.

A simple relaxation exercise is described, step by step, in Chapter 7 of this book (see p. 179).

To achieve the best results find a comfortable, warm and peaceful environment where you can sit or lie down and where there will be limited disturbance. Allow yourself enough time; at least 20 minutes once or twice a day is considered good practice. Some people like to light a candle or have some gentle aromatherapy candles or oils burning while relaxing; some like to have soft gentle sound in the background, finding that music or natural sounds can help to create an enriched relaxing environment, while for others 'silence is golden'.

Meditation Meditation can be described as the process by which we can gain awareness without thought.[50] Meditation invariably leads to a relaxed state, but it can be useful to start the process by going through a physical relaxation exercise first, to help slow the body down and release tension.

In meditation the emphasis is on stilling the mind. The body is usually positioned in an upright, balanced posture; our mind and our senses are aware of what is going on around us, but there is no interest in following sounds or distractions. The mind can be said to have moved into a more passive state of concentration, compared to the very active state of concentration and thought which we need when we are going about our daily routines.

To help us to move over from the highly thought-filled, active mind to the less active and more passive state, we can simply start off by slowing ourselves down (for example through a simple physical relaxation exercise) and then gently just starting to be aware of our breath, by gently observing the inward and outward flow – not seeking to change it, or alter it, but merely noticing it. Other ways of stilling the mind can include finding a single point of focus; this can be a sound, an image or the inner sounding of a word, softly and gently, with the voice of the mind.

The practice of meditation has extremely profound consequences. Normally our minds are full of our thoughts, feelings, emotions and sensations, and our consciousness is obscured by these. Meditation is found within many religions of the world, but it is not exclusively aligned with religion or religious practices. It is not uncommon to find that the practice of meditation highlights the importance of finding a deeper and more meaningful connection to ourselves and the underlying nature of our consciousness; it is also associated with the experience of bliss or joy, as we sense our deeper connectedness to nature and creation, whether this be framed within or outside religion. It is suggested that this consciousness is there all the time behind the habitual patterns of panic, anxiety, and preoccupation with our feelings and thoughts. An analogy helpful to many is to consider our consciousness as the blue sky that is always present behind layers of cloud. As we begin to meditate, the cloud layer gradually breaks up and we begin to see glimpses of the blue sky. The more we practise, the more of the cloud layer disappears, and every now and again the sun comes out – a moment analogous to our connecting with our higher consciousness or the divinity that is within us.

The more we practise meditation, the more we automatically go into happier, calmer, more reflective states of mind. In terms of PNI (explored in more detail in Chapter 2) we could not possibly be doing anything better for our bodies. We are effectively replacing the neuropeptide cocktail which is associated with our rather chaotic, fearful states of mind, with a beautiful, clear state in which we know very deeply that all is well and begin to understand our true relationship with life. The message that this gives to our tissues is one of profound healing.

Visualization   It has been well said that 'The power to imagine is the power to create.'[51] Visualization and guided imagery[52] have been described as a form of meditation during which you create thoughts and images, following a story with your mind's eye, and also as the conscious development and repetition of mental images which are used for a creative purpose.

The use of mind and imagination is not new to healing. After all, it is something that most of us have done at some time in our lives, starting in childhood with 'Let's pretend' or 'Let's imagine', allowing our minds to conjure up our own private pictures while listening to a story, or while being drawn into the scenes and the characters of a film or play, or in listening to music. How often have you sat down and allowed yourself to recall a happy time or event, or day-dreamed something that you hope may happen or would like to happen? Visualization and imagery are possible for all of us; we all have personal experiences, so we are already equipped to access this very special part of our healing potential. Visualization can enliven and stimulate all of our senses, not just the inner eye (mind's eye): images can include what we hear, what we smell, what we physically feel, even what we taste. All serve to connect our perceptions of our everyday outer world with the potential of the inner world, thus helping to change our reality.

The practice of visualization can show us that our perception of reality depends very much on what we think. For most of us, what we think and believe about the way things will be is an unconscious activity. This means that a great deal of what happens to us is determined by our unconscious beliefs or attitudes, and not merely what we believe about the external factors of the situations in which we find ourselves.

In the process of visualization we make conscious choices about the outcomes we want. In the context of illness this means having images of the body completely healed, images of our self strong and whole again; images of the way things will

Choosing a complementary therapist

In Appendix 2 at the back of the book you will find a list of parent organizations of the different therapeutic and self-help specialities. Many of these can give you names of qualified practitioners in your own area. It may be helpful to mention that you have cancer and want an experienced practitioner who will be confident to work with you.

If you have trouble in finding a suitable therapist, you might find some of these a useful starting point:

- your local cancer support group;
- your doctor's surgery;
- your specialist centre at hospital;
- a specialist nurse practitioner;
- health food shops;
- local complementary therapy clinics;
- friends and neighbours;
- word of mouth – often a very good source!

On finding a practitioner, remember it is your right to check with somebody what qualifications they have. If you want to make absolutely sure, you can ask for details of where they obtained their qualification and if they belong to a registered professional body. You can then obtain the telephone number of the professional body if you would like to know more about their qualifications.

Do take into consideration, however, that even though a particular practitioner might have been recommended to you, they might not be right for you, for whatever reason. Trust your intuition.

The vast majority of complementary therapists have your absolute best interests at heart. Be wary, however, of complementary therapists who make extreme claims for their interventions, or claim that you have to submit to a particular belief or philosophy in order to have the therapy.

Try not to lose heart if you need to meet one or two practitioners until you find the right one for you. Do not be pushed into making a commitment until you have experience of the therapy and therapist.

be in our life, with ourselves present at specific events in the future. We can make specific choices and goals for ourselves, which will greatly enhance the likelihood of these things coming to pass. These techniques are used in business and sports all the time, with measurable improvements in outcome.

A problem we frequently meet occurs when a doctor, who represents the voice of authority, predicts the likely outcome of an illness on the basis of statistics. This can create a very strong negative visualization, and often people who have been given a prognosis in terms of years or months to live will fulfil the prophecy almost to the day. In this situation new images, which allow for the possibility of survival and recovery, have to be created. Some people use very combative images, seeing their cancer smashed up, destroyed or attacked. Others use gentle transformative images like sun, wind, light or water, melting, dissolving, blowing or washing the illness away, seeing their body completely cleared of cancer after every visualization. (For more detailed guidance and suggestions on visualization, see Chapter 7.)

This personal visualization is different from the process of guided visualization or guided imagery in which a therapist leads you into a gentle, imaginative, pleasant frame of mind, presenting comforting, loving and beautiful images to induce a great state of well-being that produces very positive PNI changes. Experienced, psychotherapeutically trained guides use this technique to do therapeutic work with individuals or groups, to help access the emotional plane and inner wisdom.

It is also possible to use these techniques to initiate dialogue with the wounded or ill part of the self directly, asking it what is wrong and what it needs, developing in this way an extremely real relationship with the body. However, it must be stressed that this is psychotherapeutic work for which it is necessary to have a properly trained psychotherapist facilitator, so that what is brought up to consciousness can be processed and integrated for your healing.

I didn't have a great many options to recover from my tumour since I turned down orthodox medicine, but of the various alternatives offered to me visualization appealed the most because I've always believed in the power of the mind. So it was visualization that caught on with me. Then it was a question of deciding which of the different sorts of visualization I would use for my particular problem. I've always loved the sun, so that had to be involved. I relaxed each day for about two to three years, and pictured myself lying in the sun. The venue was a lovely sandy beach, with palm trees, in some far-off country. I lay on the beach listening to the sea lapping the shore. I felt the rays of the sun and felt them healing and actually shrinking the tumour. This I continued to do. I went back for various check-ups over the years, and on each occasion it was found that the tumour had shrunk. In the end there was no tumour at all – just a bit of scar tissue from the biopsy. And here I am now, and it's 12 years since I was given just a few weeks to live.

Audrey Parcell, living with inoperable lymphoma, first diagnosed in 1987

Spiritual Enquiry

Spiritual enquiry is often sparked off by the presence of serious or life-threatening illness. The kinds of questions that come to the surface are:

- What is life all about?
- Is this all there is?
- Is there a purpose to life?
- If there is a purpose, what is it and how does it affect me?
- If it is a journey, where am I going?
- Is there any sense in it all?
- What will happen to me when I die?

For centuries, millennia, people have asked these questions. All spiritual teachers tell us that often, through the very process of asking and thinking about these questions, and working on the areas of our faith, belief and understanding, the inner spiritual essence within us awakens, and with this awakening a huge amount of energy for living life in the here and now is released.

Application of the holistic approach helps us develop our spiritual awareness and consciousness, giving us a greater understanding of the whole life process. With support and healing, individuals often arrive at the belief or knowledge that they come from love and that they circle back round to love, on a great adventure of living with all its ups and downs. They know they are spiritual beings in physical bodies and that ultimately they are safe, even in death. This realization profoundly alters the whole context of life. Illness becomes a wake-up call and a time to remember who we really are spiritually; and this remembering and spiritual awakening frees us to live fully and passionately in the moment. This spiritual awakening can cause what Deepak Chopra calls 'quantum healing':[53] an acute sense of excitement, which is itself extremely healing, as great energy and joy are liberated, enabling us to experience a very great sense of aliveness and peace – even if death is quite imminent.

PART TWO
A Guide to Self-help

4

Recovering from Diagnosis and Looking Ahead

This chapter looks at what a diagnosis of cancer means and how to begin planning to cope. It covers how and where to seek advice and support, how to prepare to make choices about treatment and care, and how to set about making plans for the short- and long-term future.

Dealing with Diagnosis

The Shock

Receiving a diagnosis of cancer is probably one of the worst things we can imagine happening to us. Most of us think of it as something that happens to someone else – someone outside our family and circle of close friends. The success of modern medicine creates in us all an expectation that we will live until we are 70 or 80 years old and then die of old age. Most of us feel that good health is our birthright, and that we are basically very strong and well. So the shock of receiving the diagnosis of cancer is absolutely monumental. Nothing prepares us for this disaster: nine times out of ten there will have been hardly any build-up or warning that we are about to suffer such a devastating blow.

The effect of shock differs from person to person. But however it is felt or begins to manifest itself, the inner turmoil is such that for some time it is almost impossible to hear, let alone think clearly about, any new information that might be given. This means that an individual who has recently received a diagnosis of cancer is acutely vulnerable; and – as at any such crisis point in life – it is important to avoid, so far as possible, making any key decisions while in the state of shock.

The Reaction

The intense initial reaction to the diagnosis of cancer can take various forms. Some people collapse and give up altogether, turning their faces to the wall, living on in a state of great fear and intimidation; others attempt to submerge their feelings altogether, going into a kind of denial and trying as quickly as possible to get life 'back to normal'. For some, the immediate reaction is highly emotional, while for others the first feelings are those of complete numbness. Usually there is a period of intense disbelief, and the question 'Why me?' goes constantly round and round in the mind. It seems so random, arbitrary and unfair, and so completely out of context when you may not have felt ill at all. In many cases, the idea that a small lump, an odd-looking mole or something that has been detected by routine screening can have generated the information that one's future and very life are now critically threatened seems outrageously unbelievable and a total insult to one's sense of 'the way things are'.

Fear   For many, the initial shock quickly becomes coloured by feelings of fear, even terror. This emotion may at first have no definite form, but may then cause physical symptoms such as nausea, diarrhoea and a racing heartbeat, along with terrible panicky feelings of just not knowing how one is going to get through the next five minutes, let alone the whole day. Gradually, the feeling may become more focused, taking the form of more specifically identifiable fears – fear of pain, fear of disfigurement or disability, fear of doctors, hospitals and treatment; and, underlying this in many people's minds, the fear of death itself. Katerina Collins, who had breast cancer, said to me, 'I seriously thought I was going to die of the fear, never mind the cancer. I was even afraid to shut my eyes at night in case I died in my sleep.'

Grief   Usually very closely associated with the fear is an intense sense of grief. Often this is felt first in relation to others – children, lovers, parents, friends – because of the unbearable, searing pain at the thought of losing these people. The other major aspect of the grief is the sense of the loss of the future you thought you would have. In this very early stage it can feel almost as though you have died already, as if nothing will ever be the same again.

Relatives, too, often go into a kind of anticipatory grief. In some cases this can result in prematurely cutting themselves off from the one they love to protect themselves from the insecurity of not knowing whether he or she will live or die, be there for them or not. This feeling that friends and loved ones are withdrawing is acutely painful for the ill person, who feels abandoned with their own fear and grief.

Isolation   For whatever reason – whether it is the feeling of being put at a distance by others, jolted suddenly into contemplation of one's dying, with all the profound spiritual and existential dilemmas this creates, or the intensity of the emotions that are being experienced – what often happens next is that a strong feeling of isolation develops. This can feel like a separation from 'normal' society and 'well' colleagues – as if one has passed through an invisible local barrier to a place from which it is difficult to reach, and be reached by, others, who do not understand what is happening to you.

Within this sense of isolation can be many complicated feelings towards other people. These can include:

- jealousy, that others are living normally, not – unlike you – affected by a threat to their lives;
- resentment and anger, about the vulnerable position you are now in;
- distrust of others, fuelled by concern about becoming dependent or reliant on them, be they family or healthcare professionals;
- guilt at being a burden or a failure, at ceasing to be the provider or the emotional rock for friends or family.

The positive emotions   The other side of the picture will be the great love, closeness and gratitude that you feel as you discover friends and healthcare professionals whom you can really trust, and with whom you can allow yourself to be vulnerable and dependent.

There can also be a somewhat paradoxical phenomenon happening at the same time: for many, the shock of diagnosis, however awful, can be simultaneously tremendously energizing, triggering a period of heightened clarity and insight. In this state there can be a profound sense of stillness and truth – like being in the eye of the hurricane – so that despite the fact that your life is crashing all around you there can be a very real conviction that 'all is well' and that you really do have the inner strength to deal with the ultimate truth of the situation.

Being Real about How You Feel

The reason for spelling out these reactions in so much detail is that in Britain we tend to feel great embarrassment about our emotions. We have, in general, an abhorrence of losing control, and an inability to allow ourselves to be vulnerable or reliant in any way upon the love, care and efforts of others. This means both that individuals given a cancer diagnosis often actively suppress their reaction to the shock, and that others around them – colleagues, friends, families or health professionals – often try to get them 'back into their box' quickly, not only so that they are not embarrassing or difficult, but so that they do not cause pain to those around them.

So dominant are these tendencies that often the reaction to the diagnosis can be almost completely swept under the carpet, with people being marched straight into rigorous treatments the same day. In the attempt to keep everything as normal as possible, some people do not even stop work while undergoing chemotherapy and radiotherapy, and try in addition to maintain their normal social roles within the family and society. This pattern is echoed socially in our collective response to death itself. Frequently the bereaved are given the day off work to go to a funeral – and then it is back to 'business as usual', with no space or time whatsoever being given to accommodate the grieving and adjustment process.

At the root of all of this is the fact that as a culture we are not prepared for, or used to, the idea of disease, death and suffering. Most of us tend to live as if we were immortal, repressing and hiding that which is painful or frightening. While it is admirable that the progress of medicine has got us to this point, the failure to integrate the dying process into our lives leaves us extremely vulnerable and unprepared if we are faced with the diagnosis of life-threatening illness in ourselves or in a loved one.

Choosing Medical Treatment: Making the Right Decisions

Of course, while all this is going on there is a serious imperative to make crucial decisions about the sort of medical help you are going to have. This can be extremely difficult, especially given the complexity and diversity of medical options and protocols available for the treatment of similar cancers, and the vast array of complementary self-help and support options that exist. You may find that the Internet is helpful for you in your pursuit of information; however, be wary and try to be discerning in your search. Chrissy Holmes, the librarian at the Bristol Cancer Help Centre, has provided some very useful tips on internet resources and how to identify credible sites (see Appendix 2 for details). The confusion and difficulty this variety can generate can be even greater when healthcare professionals, because they are not fully aware of, or trained to deal with, the intense shock reaction you are going through, try to get you to make key decisions when it is almost impossible for you to think about, and take on board, what is being said.

Being Assertive

Before making these big decisions it is important not only to have clear information and be sure you have understood it, but also to feel comfortable with the course of action that has been recommended to you, and to be clear as to how you are going to go about dealing with the problem that now faces you.

Assertiveness is not the same thing as aggression. Many of us fear being judged aggressive if we assert ourselves, and therefore do not speak out for our own needs; as a result we end up feeling frustrated and unheard. But being assertive does not mean being aggressive; what it does mean is asking directly and openly for your needs to be heard and respected. This is your body, and you have a right to the major say in what happens to it. Medical terms may be used that you do not understand and need to have explained. There may be more details of the side-effects, or effectiveness, of the treatment options on offer to be discussed. You may need to ask for time to think about your next steps.

When being assertive it is helpful to have a clear idea what you are asking for, couch the request in simple terms, and keep repeating the same sentence until you feel it has been respond-ed to. Examples might be:

- 'I would like more time to think about this.'
- 'Could you please explain . . . again?'
- 'I have always used natural medicine, the idea of chemotherapy is difficult for me.'
- 'Could you tell me a little more about possible side-effects?'

Seeking Clear Information

Another issue that strongly affects your ability to make impor-tant decisions is the clarity of the picture of your problem you are given. Sometimes cancer healthcare professionals will with-hold information on the recommendation of relatives, or will themselves choose to water down what they tell you in order to protect you emotionally. This is quite understandable, but can create a false impression. On the other hand, they can make the power of conventional medicine to treat or cure cancer sound stronger than it is. Statistics on the potential of treatments to improve survival may actually reflect only the potential to increase the 'disease-free interval' (the period of time during which you will not be bothered by symptoms or obvious mani-festations of the disease). Again, it is totally understandable that healthcare professionals should wish to give as upbeat a picture as possible; but clarity is very important if you are to make sound decisions. This question of how completely realis-tic you wish to be about the 'bottom line' lies very much in your own hands; your doctors and nurses will often be looking for cues from you about how much you wish to know. Ideally, you will be able to say directly to them exactly how much you can deal with on each occasion you see them.

Remember, if you are given bad news, that a statistic is *not* a certainty. Statistics do not take into consideration an individ-ual's response to a situation. As has already been discussed in

Chapter 2 on the scientific evidence, there is a whole variety of strategies that can be utilized to enhance your potential for recovery. If you feel your body is in a state of shock after a diagnosis, or if you feel that the bad news you have received has become embedded in your mind, it may well be helpful for you to seek out support from a counsellor or hypnotherapist. It will be important for you to regain a sense of hope regarding your situation – whatever that may mean for you in your own individual situation.

Planning a Visit to Your Doctor to Discuss Treatments

Always try to have a good friend or family member with you at any consultation, even if you think it will be a routine visit, as a kind of 'advocate': that is, someone who will be able to remember what is said and will support you in making sure your questions are answered.

Be prepared, too, to ask for more time to consider questions that are put to you; you should not be rushed into anything. Here again it may well help to have a supportive companion with you.

Consider taking a tape-recorder to tape the session so you don't forget any of the content of the conversation. This also gives you the opportunity to listen to the options slowly at home, to formulate further questions, and to share the information with family or friends.

Don't be afraid to ask questions or ask to look at notes, results of tests or observations. Think of the questions you want to ask before you go. If you know what your questions are in advance, do write them down to remind yourself, as the consultation may be stressful and it can be easy to forget.

It is quite in order to personalize any questions you ask; for example, if you want to, ask your doctor, 'If you were me, what would you do in this situation?'

As an example of the kinds of things you might think about, here are some suggested questions you might ask if you were trying to consider a particular type of treatment that had been offered:

- Would *you* take this treatment if it were offered to you?
- What is the usual course of the disease both with and without this treatment?
- What are the side-effects of this treatment?
- What are the available alternatives to this treatment?
- Do the benefits of having the treatment outweigh the risks?
- How will this treatment affect, for better or for worse, my quality of life?
- Are there any new treatments, or trials of new treatments, for my particular condition happening in the UK?

It is also worth reflecting on how you will cope with the answers you may get to your questions. Doctors get a lot of their information from statistics, and are used to presenting possibilities in statistical terms. Do remember, however, that statistics deal with trends, not with individuals' particular responses to treatment; everyone's disease behaves differently. Statistics can give you valuable contextual information and help you to weigh possibilities, but they do not tell you *what will happen*.

Do remember that you have the right to take a second opinion if you wish. This option is discussed later in the chapter in the section on 'Medical Information' (see pp. 113–15). If you wish to investigate this option, contact your GP in the first instance.

Taking the Time You Need

Because it is likely that others around you may fail to recognize and make adjustments for the state you are in, it becomes doubly important that you do so. This applies not only at the time of primary diagnosis but also if recurrences are diagnosed; then the impact can be even worse than it was the first time around. There can also be points of key vulnerability when your medical treatment stops and you are suddenly left to face the reality of your situation alone, without the framework provided by the care of your medical team and the focus and rigours of your treatment process.

In recognizing perhaps just how shocked or upset you are, at all or any of these moments, your primary need will probably be for time:

- time to take on board what has happened;
- time to feel, express and process your feelings;
- time to think about medical decision-making processes;
- time to get the relevant information you need;
- time to think about how the diagnosis will affect your life and the lives of those close to you;
- time to think about whom you want to tell, and how;
- time for all the planning for change that diagnosis and treatment will demand.

When you have had time to consider all the factors that apply in your case, you may need to claim time over the longer term:

- If you are about to embark on a course of treatment, it is very possible that you will need to take leave of absence from work and regular social commitments, during which you may need to arrange cover for your family and your colleagues.
- You may well need a good old-fashioned period of convalescence during and after your treatment so that you can recover fully before going back to work, if going back to work at all is appropriate in the bigger picture.

Above all, try very hard to let go of feelings of duty to others during this period. It is very important that you put yourself right at the top of the list of people you look after, and indeed this may be an essential part of what you need to do over the long term for your deeper healing process. The period during which you are ill, or in shock, or receiving treatment, is a very good opportunity to get used to doing this.

Embarking on Treatment

Within the world of mainstream cancer medicine, things usually start to happen the minute a diagnosis of cancer is made. Many of the people who come to the Bristol Cancer Help Centre describe this immediate-action response to their diagnosis as 'like being hit by a steam train'. Often, within a single conversation, an individual is given the diagnosis and prognosis, and then presented with a complex array of surgical, chemotherapeutic and radiotherapeutic options – and then, not infrequently, asked to make a choice from the list and give consent for treatments to begin: all at the same time, when the individual is in a state of profound shock and distress.

Studies have shown repeatedly that during that first conversation, from the moment the word 'cancer' is uttered, people hardly ever retain a single other word that is said. This means that, more often than not, consent for treatments to be implemented is being elicited during conversations that people don't even recall. Not only is no time allowed for the person to absorb the shock, no time is made available before treatments are embarked upon for the intense emotional reaction that follows diagnosis, or for any support to be given. This means that individuals are usually starting treatment in not the best frame of mind: full of emotion, and without either genuinely understanding what is happening to them or having given truly informed consent.

There are many times when having medical treatment is the right thing to do, but if at all possible this should take place only when an individual has had sufficient chance to recover from the shock and upset of diagnosis, and he or she is able to hear and properly understand what is being said by others. This is important, even if it means that key medical information has to be repeated many times.

The key here is to insist that medical personnel allow you sufficient time to think about the major decisions involving treatment and care, so that you can become adjusted, motivated, properly prepared and, ultimately, strongly committed to a particular course of action. Whatever else happens, it is vital to make sure that you are not being rushed, even if it seems to some that you are being slow and obstinate. Remember that the medical profession is there to serve your needs and not the other way around. Don't be afraid to ask your specialist to draw diagrams or use simpler explanations, so that you can understand what he or she plans to do.

Ideally, treatment should not be commenced until truly informed consent has been obtained, and the individual feels confident and right about the treatment being undertaken. Often our own intuition or inner wisdom knows what is best for us as an individual, and in an ideal world you would ask for, and be able to listen to, its advice as to which approach is correct for you; but this is usually more easily said than done when you are in shock, feeling pressurized and most likely afraid and confused. Nevertheless, your 'gut feeling' about treatment should be heeded, explored and very possibly followed. A doctor who is familiar with the holistic approach, such as those at the Centre, can help you to contact your intuition and include its input in the decision process. If positive associations and feelings towards the treatment have been developed before the treatment starts, this is good, as the individual does not then embark on it while harbouring the very frightening, negative images that many people have in connection with chemotherapy and radiotherapy.

An Integrated Approach: Combining Mainstream and Holistic Therapy

By combining holistic and mainstream therapies you can support your body's system to help combat the downside of conventional interventions, most especially in helping to repair damage to healthy tissue straight away.

Many proponents of alternative therapies insist that people will have far better outcomes if they use natural medicines alone. However, this view places the individual with cancer under acute pressure to decide 'which camp to join'. The decision to use one model of therapy in preference to another must be thought about carefully and taken on an absolutely individual basis. In cases in which the cancer is low-grade and in its early stages, the individual has time on their side and may therefore opt to work with alternative approaches alone for a period and then judge for themselves whether or not they are achieving stabilization or regression of their disease.

In other situations there may be a time imperative – in cases where there is a possibility of a tumour's becoming inoperable, for example, or posing a threat locally to nervous or arterial tissue. In such cases, urgent medical intervention may be required to save life or prevent disability. It may also be advisable to remove a tumour if there is a risk that it will break through the skin and develop into a nasty, ulcerating lesion. The best course of action for those faced with this dilemma is to talk to a holistic doctor, who will help you to evaluate realistically which option or combination of options would be best for you when all the various factors and personal views are taken into consideration. In this way, it is hoped that you will be able to decide on a course of action that both honours your personal needs and keeps you as safe as possible.

The Doctors at the Bristol Cancer Help Centre

The doctors at the Centre have specialized in an integrated

approach to the care of people with cancer and have a good working knowledge of mainstream medicine; thus they are able to act as a bridge, understanding the values of a combination of both approaches.

The decision-making process is one of the areas in which these doctors can be very useful. The first thing they do is to review the medical situation of each individual, taking time to explain exactly what is going on medically and what the treatments offered involve. They will compare these with other options that may be available, and look fully at the possible implications of not having treatment, if this is an option you are considering. Often, time with these doctors can help an individual formulate – and develop the confidence to ask – the key questions to be addressed during subsequent medical consultations.

This process of review is important, particularly for those people who have, as an immediate reaction, flatly refused any medical treatment when in fact at least some surgical intervention may well prevent disagreeable complications. On the other hand, saying no to treatment may be the wiser option if the disease is very advanced and treatments can realistically promise only very minor improvement with a great loss of quality of life, and if sufficient inner strength can be cultivated to enable the individual to cope without treatment.

Getting What You Need – and Going On Getting It

This issue of taking charge does not apply only to the decision-making process with regard to treatments. It is very important that you take, and retain, similar control during all your interactions with the medical profession. Believe it or not, after the scientific study that showed that 'difficult' patients live longer, one support group in America had T-shirts printed with the legend 'I am a difficult patient' for people to wear on their trips to hospital.

By and large the British tend to be very passive in the face of authority, and to cherish a belief in the power of the medical profession to take care of us and sort everything out if we become ill. For many people, the cancer diagnosis is their first experience of the medical system outside the GP's surgery. As daunting as it may seem, it can be useful to step back from the advice that you receive from your own particular hospital consultant or unit and, if you are able to, try to look at what is going on in the bigger picture, not just nationally but worldwide, with respect to your type of cancer. Advances in conventional treatment continue to be made; so, ideally, you should make sure that you are fully aware of all the current treatments and that there are no other options you could be exploring. The ways in which you can go about collecting this kind of information are discussed in the Medical Information section later in this chapter (see pp. 113–15).

It is even more important, and perhaps even harder, to absorb soon after diagnosis the fact that cancer medicine does not currently have all the answers. This means that what the medical profession has to offer, which is extremely important in controlling the unpleasant manifestations of the disease, should be viewed realistically – as one part of your holistic cancer plan; it should definitely not be passively relied upon to get you better.

Ideally, you should be striving for the best possible medical treatment with the highest possible degree of individualization of your care. This means ensuring that:

- You are given time to recover from the shock of diagnosis or bad news before being expected to think about treatment decisions.
- Treatment decisions are made with reference to all the relevant information (having consulted several sources).
- Your needs for support and counselling throughout the processes have been provided for; if the medical unit that

you are dealing with does not have facilities for this, they should direct you to organizations, local or national, who can help.

- You have been advised about other support agencies relevant to your particular illness or its treatment; you may not want to use them now, but they may come in handy in the future.
- Prior to making decisions on medical treatment, you have access to information about the full range of alternative, complementary and mind–body options available in Britain and abroad, with (if possible) guidance on their use.

Communicating with Healthcare Professionals

The main thing that will make a difference to whether or not you get what you want is how well you are able to communicate with healthcare professionals, namely your consultant, your GP and key nursing staff. This in turn will depend upon the openness and preparedness of medical personnel to take your views on board and to cater to your needs. It will help you to know that in the policy framework for commissioning cancer services – formulated by Drs Calman and Hine, and known as the Calman–Hine Report of 1995 – the second of the key recommendations and action points is:

The needs of patients and their carers should be the primary concern of purchasers, planners and professionals involved in cancer services.

The fourth of seven key principles that should govern the provision of cancer care is that:

the development of cancer services should be patient-centred and should take account of patients', families' and carers' views and preferences as well as those of professionals involved in cancer care. Individuals' perceptions of their needs may differ from those of the professional. Good communication between professionals and patients is especially important.

If you are not sure how your team should be helping to establish, and provide for, your needs, it is worth consulting the Calman–Hine Report, which outlines good practice. The report is a Department of Health document and should be available from public libraries.

More recently, in 2000 the NHS published *The NHS Cancer Plan*, setting out the first ever comprehensive government strategy to tackle cancer: a major programme of action covering prevention, diagnosis, treatment, care and research. The document can be found on the Internet at www.doh.gov.uk/cancer, or you can get it by post, free of charge, from the Department of Health, PO Box 777, London SE1 6XH.

Setting Up Your Support Network

After recognizing your needs for time and information, the thing you will next need to recognize is your need for support. As noted earlier in this chapter, most of us are very resistant to the idea of asking for help: we find it embarrassing or humiliating, and we hate the feeling of being 'out of control' or indebted to others. Quite often these feelings are rooted in a fear of intimacy or low self-esteem: we might consider ourselves unworthy of the time and attention of others, feeling that we must pay back anything that is given to us, or we might feel shame at appearing vulnerable emotionally or physically. It is deeply sad that our culture has had this effect on us. The most powerful need in all human beings is for a sense of connection with one another in order that we may give and receive love. Indeed, very often, providing the opportunity for others to give is – far from being a burden – a gift for them. Just ask yourself which gives you the better feeling: receiving or giving?

Many have said how they wished that healing could be a nice straightforward affair, after which one could carry on life as before. But, in the immortal words of Penny Brohn, 'healing is a process, not an event', and the different parts of the healing process go on at different levels at different rates. It is therefore important to remain open to this healing process even when you feel inclined to close the book and try not to think about it. At times, the way forward will be clear, but at others it will be obscure. This is why it is wise to organize as much support as possible, so that you can draw on it when you lose the plot and need help, encouragement and guidance.

Spreading the Work of Support

Frequently, though, the problem is that people are not clear enough about the fact that they are in distress and need help – or about the kind of help they need. Most often, to avoid feelings of dependency and embarrassment, people turn to the individual to whom they are closest, be that a friend, relative or partner. This is totally natural, but has certain inherent problems. First of all, your relationship with that person will become dominated by the illness. Second, any existing tensions or weaknesses in the relationship will be exaggerated, maybe critically. The last thing you need is a key relationship crumbling at a time when you are most vulnerable, and certainly the intense needs associated with illness and its treatment are not a particularly good way to try to test, improve or revive a difficult relationship. The third reason is that if most of your distress is being mopped up by the person closest to you, this will almost inevitably, directly or indirectly, rebound on you in some way, in much the same way as a pinball ricochets backwards and forwards within the pinball machine's closed system. In close relationships or family systems the distress ricochets around, affecting first one and then another member of the family or network – until it comes back to you, perhaps in a different form, especially if you are usually the main carer in the family.

It is therefore important to build for yourself a support system that is large enough for the purpose right from the start. This means including sufficient people to spread the load and prevent the team going into 'support fatigue'.

Who to Include in Your Support Team

Ideally, the team should be made up of individuals who are sufficiently well supported in their own lives to be able to give what they can without any sense on either side of debt or payback. Try to sit down and, in a very organized way, think of a dozen or so people whom you can invite to be part of your support team, asking them explicitly if they can be 'there for you' in one way or another if you need them. This means that when help becomes essential, you already have your support network in place. Having a very real team like this also makes it far less likely that your close carer will sink without trace under the stress and distress they are feeling. In fact, if the main support and care are coming from your support team, personal and professional, and your partner, too, finds ways of getting the necessary support and care, there is a genuine chance that the time with your nearest and dearest can be spent in having fun rather than in attempting to counsel and support each other.

In addition to friends and loved ones, the support team may well include professional people, such as counsellors, specialist nurses, social workers, ministers and the team of therapists you find to help you; it may also include members of cancer support groups you meet locally or through the Bristol Cancer Help Centre. Certainly if this issue is addressed head-on, and support is organized actively, it will make an enormous difference in planning for and dealing with what has to be faced on a day-to-day basis.

Some people have gone so far as to form their support team into a personal support group of friends who meet on a regular basis so that all members can hear about what is going on and what support is needed. This does not have to be a one-way process: it can also be an opportunity for you to listen to what is happening for them, too; and this in itself can be very empowering all round because, as their needs will probably differ from yours, the insight you are gaining through your own process of living with the illness may be of immense value to them.

How It Can Work

An excellent example of how a support team can work is given in the story of Veronica Mills, who came to the Centre in the early 1980s. She had gone to have a mole removed from her chin for cosmetic reasons when it was discovered that the mole was a melanoma. She was told that there were serious metastases in her liver and that she had only three months to live. She was utterly determined that this would not be the case, especially since she had only recently adopted two children. In fact, she lived for over nine years from the time of her diagnosis – until both children were out of school. Very early on in the weeks that followed her diagnosis, she realized that nearly all of her friends had stopped telephoning her, and she sensed that they were completely at a loss as to what to say or how to help. With extraordinary resolution and clear-sightedness, she wrote a letter to everyone she knew, beginning:

Dear Friend,
    Yes, I have cancer. Yes, I have been told I have only three months left to live – but actually I am still here! And I need:

1   Flowers every week.
2   Somebody to pick up my organic vegetables each week.
3   Money for my holistic therapy.
4   Somebody to take my children out while I meditate and
    visualize.
5   A holiday in the Bahamas.
6   Any information any of you can find about alternative
    treatment for cancer anywhere in the world . . .

. . . and her list went on and on, detailing about 20 practical ways in which people could help her. Veronica got absolutely every single thing on her list – and more – along with letters of intense gratitude from the people who loved her saying, 'Thank God you told us what we could do to help. We were aching to do something but didn't have a clue what would make a difference.'

Veronica's approach was exceptionally up-front, but it beautifully illustrates the point that for most of us there is probably a great deal more help available within our social network than we would ever imagine: all we have to do is become clear about what it is that we need, and then let go of our inhibitions and ask for it – and, of course, be prepared for the answer 'No' if somebody recognizes that at this point they are not in a position to help. And that is quite all right too.

Where to Seek Support

If you do not have strong personal social networks, it is all the more important to get yourself to cancer support groups or local community groups like your church, a yoga class, or anywhere where kind, loving people meet, and make your need known. One of the loveliest things that people have said about the Bristol Cancer Help Centre over the years is, 'We could not believe the incredible amount of love we received from total strangers.' This emphasizes even more strongly the point that, sometimes, stepping out of one's family and social network can open up the possibility of receiving help from sources you never even imagined were there, and indeed enriching the lives of others by giving them the opportunity to be helpful and to express their care.

Along with finding sources of support, get really practical and, like Veronica, make a list of absolutely everything you need. Then begin asking – either directly or by letter – for the items on the list. Having your list worked out also means that when friends spontaneously offer help, you do not waste the golden opportunity: you will be prepared and will know exactly what to ask for. You will find very quickly that with a little bit of practice the embarrassment goes and it starts to feel quite natural.

While you're at it, ask your family what they need. In this way you can short-circuit any problem of growing resentment as they begin to see the things you have asked for flowing towards you!

Finding the Information You Need

If you can follow the guidelines set out in this chapter about ensuring that you have space and time to take your own decisions, and an adequate level of support, this will make it much easier to begin the process of taking control of your situation. This process usually starts with gathering information and seeing what choices you have in terms of how you tackle your cancer and the emotional upheaval it has caused.

The information you will need falls into four main categories:

- medical information about your condition and its treatment;
- information about complementary, alternative and self-help approaches;
- information about support services;
- practical information about how the cancer services operate in your area.

(You will find some relevant telephone numbers and contact addresses relating to this section in Appendix 2.)

Medical Information
The best agency in Britain dealing with medical information about cancer and its treatment is CancerBACUP (formerly

BACUP, the British Association of Cancer Unit Patients). CancerBACUP has an extensive range of leaflets about all types of cancer and their treatment, and a telephone helpline to answer more specific questions. This can be very useful if you find your own medical team have not given you enough time to ask all the questions you need to ask. It can also be a lot less daunting than medical libraries, where information is written up in very stark terminology, which can be alienating and frightening because it has been written for those treating, rather than experiencing, cancer.

What you will probably not get from CancerBACUP is information about pioneering techniques or experimental clinical trials, which may be happening at the cutting edge of medicine. It can be very useful to try to track down who is leading the field in your particular kind of cancer. This can usually be discovered by talking to medical personnel in your oncology centre, or by phoning the colleges of the particular disciplines involved. The other source of this information is Cancer Research UK, the biggest British cancer charity.

Having gathered this information, you may then wish to compare it with what is going on in America. Here the first step may be to contact the American Cancer Society, which will be able to point you towards leaders in the field in America. The Sloan-Kettering Memorial Hospital in New York is another good source of information about American advances. All of these organizations have information departments, with usually very helpful staff. There is, of course, also the Internet (see Appendix 2); but the problem here is dealing with the huge quantity and complexity of the information that you are likely to find. Nevertheless, it may be a good way to follow up the information you are getting from the various sources, and begin to see which way the path is leading.

It is important to find out from the hospital cancer service, your GP, health visitors and the nursing support services exactly what facilities and services are available to you: through the

Seeking a second opinion

It is usually possible to get a second opinion on the NHS. If you discover that there are better treatments for your condition in parts of the country other than your own health authority area, you may be able to negotiate help from outside your own area. However, in practice, this means that the degree of success that you have in obtaining help from elsewhere often reflects the amount of detective work you are prepared to put in, and the assertiveness with which you pursue other avenues of help. While it is unacceptable that there should be such a degree of demographical variation in standards and knowledge available, it is the reality of the situation, and we are therefore obliged to take account of it.

NHS and through the voluntary sector, locally and throughout the country. People with cancer often complain that they only discovered much later about valuable local services that they would have used if they'd known about them. There may also be many practical ways you could be receiving help, financially, socially and emotionally. Many cancer centres and units are in the process of building good information units; you may be lucky and find that your own treatment centre has both the information and somebody there who can lead you through it.

Once you have gathered the information you need, you may wish to return to discuss it with your consultant, or to seek a second opinion with whoever it is you have discovered is leading the field in the speciality that relates to you (see box).

Complementary and Self-help Approaches

It is hoped that your need for information about the holistic approach to cancer will have been met at least in part by reading this book or watching the Bristol Cancer Help Centre's video, *The Holistic Approach to Health*. In either case, it will be abundantly clear that it is necessary to address the psychospiritual components of your illness as well as the physical.

Bear in mind that not all alternative medical treatments take into account the underlying state of spirit and mind which is crucial to immune functioning in the longer term. It may therefore be necessary for you to organize the mind–body aspect of your approach separately, in addition to any alternative treatment you decide to use as part of your overall plan.

As with the medical information, when you have investigated all the alternative and complementary options you may be somewhat overwhelmed by the diversity of what you have discovered. It may be wise at this point to seek an appointment with a doctor who you feel understands the integrated approach and who can help you to consider all the options and work out which one is the most suitable for you, including the possibility of a course at Bristol.

Support Services

Britain has a number of support groups and centres that have been developed by people who have used the Bristol Approach (details of these are available from the Centre; see Appendix 2 for contact details). These groups are absolutely ideal for those who would like to use the Bristol Approach, as they offer support in finding the right kind of therapists, learning the self-help techniques, and maintaining a strong positive attitude. In addition to these, there are hundreds of further support groups around Britain, which are held in a directory by Macmillan Cancerlink. In addition to these there are disease- and problem-specific support groups, which should be known to your cancer centre/unit information service or to Macmillan Cancerlink. Macmillan has recently produced a *Directory of Complementary Therapy Services in UK Cancer Care*, which can be obtained by telephoning the number given in Appendix 2.

Other kinds of support agencies include those that deal with legal, financial, social and nursing care needs. Again, these should be known to your cancer unit/centre, but if not, ring the

Bristol Cancer Help Centre's national telephone helpline: 0117 980 9505.

Your Local Cancer Services

It may serve you very well at difficult moments to know exactly how the cancer services operate in your area, so it is worth finding out all you can as soon as possible, for example:

- the management structure and overall policy for your area;
- what facilities and practical help are available;
- what support and complementary services are provided, and what the attitude is regarding these services in your area;
- how to access the help of specialist nurses – e.g. Macmillan, Marie Curie or the local community nurse – and what role your GP will play in this;
- how to access specialist pain control;
- how to get a second opinion or referral to a specialist hospital, such as an NHS homoeopathic hospital;
- if there is a local hospice (you may wish to visit);
- if your GP is allowed to prescribe you vitamins;
- if your area health authority provides complementary therapies routinely, or will pay for alternative treatment if your conventional treatment is no longer working.

Nowadays Macmillan nurses can be involved from the onset and can be an invaluable source of support, both practical and psychological. They may also be able to inform you about financial entitlements or other available funding.

Some of this information will be available from the information centre at the hospital where you are being treated; some will be available from your GP or local primary care group committee, and some from the local headquarters of the nursing services. If you are not getting the answers you need, or feel concerned about what you are discovering, you should contact the director or manager of cancer services for your area through your local cancer centre/unit or health authority.

Moving On

Once you have sifted through the information and made informed choices, you can embark on the treatments you have chosen in the empowering knowledge that the medical help you are receiving is one part of a much bigger picture that you now see clearly. You will, it is hoped, have taken on board that you can be as powerful an agent in your own defence as the medical treatment that is being offered to you, and that even if there is no medical treatment on offer there are many very significant steps you can take to increase the possibility of living with cancer.

5
Coping with Treatment

This chapter suggests how you can draw on the therapies, complementary medicines and self-help techniques used at the Bristol Centre to:

- help you prepare for medical treatment;
- alleviate cancer-related symptoms;
- moderate the side-effects of treatment.

Using the Bristol Approach in Preparation for Treatment

There is now a large amount of evidence to suggest that many of the therapies and self-healing techniques employed at Bristol can be very effective in reducing both the side-effects of treatment and general cancer-related symptoms. Indeed, they come into their own before any treatment actually gets under way; for it is vitally important that you are adequately prepared, psychologically and physically, for any treatment you may undergo.

This preparation may include obtaining relevant information about your illness and the available treatments, as explored in the previous chapter. You may also find that using relaxation therapy, meditation and visualization (as described in Chapter 7) helps to minimize the degree of distress involved. This broad approach[54] has been shown to significantly reduce side-effects and the risk of post-treatment complications, while simultaneously improving treatment toleration and even the chances of survival.

Physical Preparation: Diet and Nutrition

A great deal can also be done to prepare yourself physically, particularly through attention to diet. All conventional treatments – surgical, chemotherapeutic and radiotherapeutic – are tolerated better if you are in a good state nutritionally. Those who have embarked upon chemotherapy or radiotherapy both before and after adopting a healthy diet say that the difference is remarkable. When the body is in a less toxic state, the toxicity of these treatments seems often to be better tolerated. Good nutrition is also extremely helpful in preparing the body for surgery. Most surgical procedures involve a period before the operation of having nothing to eat – 'nil by mouth' – and of course an extended period of recovery afterwards when sometimes the appetite is low or it is difficult to eat. To help your body cope with this, vitamin and mineral supplementation should ideally start immediately after diagnosis, as should any other improvements you can make in diet to prepare the ground. (For the Bristol Cancer Help Centre's guidelines on nutrition, see Appendix 1.)

Emotional Preparation and Monitoring

Your emotional state should also be considered throughout the treatment process. The treatment itself can produce depression or anxiety, and this may build up over time. This, coupled with exhaustion and/or physical side-effects, may mean that you become too vulnerable to receive a session of treatment at the proposed time; at this point you may need to ask for some extra support or recovery time before continuing with treatment. It is

important that both you and the healthcare professionals working with you recognize this possibility and are sensitive to your
needs. People who do not acknowledge their own sense of vulnerability, or who ignore their inner voice saying 'Stop' and continue with treatment when they know they cannot cope with it,
may find themselves in a psychological or physical crisis.

Key Points to Assist You in Preparing for Treatment
- Ensure you have all the relevant information you need.
- Build up your body's energy levels and health by giving it
  the best nourishment you can (see Appendix 1).
- Send off for the Bristol Cancer Help Centre's guidelines on
  vitamins, 'The Bristol Approach to Nutrition and
  Supplements'.
- Find someone to whom you can express your fears and
  any concerns you have about treatment. This may be
  more easily done with someone who is not a family
  member or friend.
- If you have the opportunity, find a counsellor or relaxation
  therapist who can teach you some relaxation, meditation
  or visualization techniques; alternatively, buy a selection of
  self-help guides from the Centre's mail order catalogue or
  from a local bookshop (many now have 'Mind/Body/Spirit'
  sections).

Support during Periods in Hospital

Nurturing the Senses . . .
When you go into hospital, take things that will nurture *all*
your physical senses. For example:

- *Sight* – inspiring photos or cards, beautiful flowers.
- *Sound* – relaxing music tapes, relaxation tapes, talking
  books (don't forget the personal stereo or CD player!).

- *Smell* – aromotherapy oils. Just a few drops on a tissue can be very effective: lavender is relaxing, reduces nausea and headaches and helps promote restful sleep; bergamot is pleasantly stimulating. (But note that care needs to be taken with some aromatherapy oils if you are receiving chemotherapy; discuss this with your care team.)
- *Touch* – a soft nightshirt, cuddly toy, little blanket or soft pillow.
- *Taste* – healthy light foods or drinks you enjoy.

. . . and the Sense of Humour
Essential!

- Encourage friends who make you laugh to visit.
- Take, or get people to bring or send you, funny videos, books, cartoons and emails.

Practising Self-help Techniques in Hospital
The self-help techniques of relaxation, meditation and visualization, described in more detail in Chapter 7, can be effectively used during a stay in hospital, or when visiting the hospital departments for daily treatment. Hospital staff can give you more support if you let them know what you are doing; so tell them, for example, if you need a few minutes to settle yourself to listen to a personal audio tape or CD to help you to relax or visualize, or listen to calming music. Let them know, too, if you want to practise any of these techniques before chemotherapy or radiotherapy, or indeed any other procedure; it can provide help and insight for them as well as helping you to cope better.

A hospital, of course, can be a less than ideal environment in which to practise these techniques. You may find there is noise around you, and sometimes a lack of privacy creates distractions. You may well find it easier if you have established a habit of practising at home first – another strand of your preparation! Even so, once in hospital you might not be able to motivate yourself to perform a personal visualization or relaxation; maybe your mind is too full of worrying thoughts or preoccupations, or just not able to settle down enough to get the full benefit from the technique. This would be one time when you might benefit more from a prepared tape or CD on a personal audio-cassette or CD player – preferably with individual earphones – so that you can just listen and follow the exercises peacefully.

Therapies and Techniques to Support Yourself During Treatment

Complementary therapies and self-help techniques can be used in conjunction with orthodox treatment, though care needs to be taken with some aromatherapy oils if you are receiving chemotherapy, and it is important that your medical team are informed as to which therapies you are using. Techniques such as meditation and visualization can be used to promote a relaxation response in the body and can also be used proactively to support you through treatment.

Visualization and Relaxation
Visualize all treatments as very effective, doing their job and not interfering with the rest of the body. See repair to full health being rapid and easy. Visualize rays of your radiotherapy as rays of the sun warming, soothing and healing your body. Chemotherapy could be envisaged as the elixir of life, coursing through your body and ridding it of any unwanted, damaged cells. These images can make the experience of these treatments more positive and manageable.

Research has shown that using visualization and relaxation techniques can:

- increase one's sense of control;[55]
- lower stress, anxiety and depression;[56]

- reduce nausea and pain;[57] and
- improve immunological function.[58]

Bodywork

The use of energy-based therapies such as reflexology, acupuncture and shiatsu can all help reduce physical symptoms as well as enhance the energy flow throughout the body, which improves well-being and the body's ability to heal. Massage and aromatherapy massage can enable release of both physical and mental tension, so:

- relieving pain;[59]
- reducing anxiety and improving sleep.[60]

Mind–Body–Spirit Work

Spiritual healing can also be an opportunity to give time to yourself and honour your physical, emotional and spiritual needs. The healer may be able to help with visualization and meditation practice, and will also be able to balance energy in your body, promote relaxation and strengthen the spirit.

The mind–body connection is extremely strong. When you recognize this, come to understand the way in which it operates (see Chapter 2 and Chapter 7) and begin to work with it in daily life, the effects can be very powerful.

Managing Your Symptoms

The Three Sides of Symptoms

Symptoms invariably have three components (although all these are, of course, interlinked):

- the physical aspect of the symptom;
- the emotional response to the symptom, which if not addressed may exacerbate it;

- the spiritual dimension of the symptom, which embraces the background, culture, work and home life and social activities of the individual, and acknowledges the uniqueness of each person in their response to situations and symptoms.

Complementary symptom management is therefore usually directed at addressing each of these levels.

Complementary Symptom Management

Techniques such as muscle relaxation, visualization and meditation, bodywork therapies such as massage and shiatsu, as well as aromatherapy and breathing techniques, can all be used to help relax the mind and body and thereby have a direct influence on the unconscious processes of the body, helping them to function more efficiently. Specific therapies, such as acupuncture, reflexology, homoeopathic and herbal remedies can be used to manage the physical aspects of the symptoms and strengthen the body's innate power to self-heal (see Chapter 3 for an overiew of these therapies and techniques).

Complementary therapies and relaxation techniques can be very comforting and help facilitate the expression of emotions. They may lead to an emotional catharsis, in turn generating a greater acceptance of the situation. Though many of the techniques can be self-taught and used independently, the process can be facilitated by a therapist with whom you build an empathic bond and with whom you feel safe to 'let go'. Often, the degree to which symptoms are reduced as a result of relaxation and emotional expression and understanding is so great that either the symptom becomes entirely manageable or it can be controlled by natural remedies or reduced levels of conventional drugs. Note, however, that we are *not* suggesting you give up your conventional medication; it is recognized that medication can play an invaluable role in the control of symptoms.

At the Bristol Cancer Help Centre an assessment is made for each individual of the nature of the symptoms and their causes so that appropriate therapies and techniques can be offered. If you do not come to the Centre, however, you may find the ideas below helpful. These next few sections suggest therapies and techniques that may be used to control or alleviate specific symptoms.

Anxiety/Insomnia

Aromatherapy   Ideally, seek out an aromatherapist who can recommend specific oils for your individual situation. Otherwise the following oils may be helpful:

- lavender — as a sedative, calming oil;
- frankincense — helps relaxation by deepening the breathing;
- neroli — helps with anxiety;
- ylang ylang — helps with feelings of frustration and depression;
- rose — queen of oils, soothing and anti-depressant.

Bach Flower Remedies   These essences work on the emotional level. They were developed from flowers by Dr Edward Bach, a pathologist and bacteriologist, in the early twentieth century. The therapy is based on the premiss that disease is directly linked to temperament; the remedies were designed to assist people to manage their emotions/temperament more effectively. Bach developed 38 essences in all, of which the following may be particularly helpful for anxiety and insomnia:

- white chestnut — persistent worrying thoughts;
- elm — feeling overwhelmed and unable to cope;
- mimulus — for fear;
- star of Bethlehem — when still in shock;
- rock rose — for general calming.

Relaxation and breathing   See Chapter 7 for a detailed description of a specific relaxation exercise.

Other useful aids to assist sleeping
• Valerian (a herbal remedy easily obtained from most health food shops).
• Gentle foot, face or hand massage.
• Sleep cones – these plastic cones, which can be found in natural health food shops, can be applied to an acupuncture point to help induce sleep.
• Listening to soothing music.
• Listening to relaxation tapes.
• Homoeopathy.
• Acupuncture.
• Yoga/tai chi.
• Taking a short walk outdoors before you lie down to sleep.

Taking a 'cat nap' or a period where you lie down and allow yourself to relax or sleep during the day will help you to cope better with treatments.

Ensure that you exclude unnecessary light from the room in which you sleep; this might otherwise prevent you from going into a deep sleep.

Pain
Breathing exercises   When in pain we tend to hold our breath or breathe in a shallow and rapid way, which makes us more receptive and sensitive to pain. When we change the breathing pattern, breathing more deeply and slowly, the body responds by relaxing the muscles. Focusing on the breath can also act as a distraction from the pain.

Visualization   This is a powerful self-help tool which is described in detail in Chapter 7. At first it might be difficult to do, but techniques to help you to visualize or imagine the pain can help to reduce it or give you more control over it. One approach would be to think about the size, shape, colour and voice of the pain, so bringing consciousness to it. This can transform or reduce the symptom and may, in addition, provide meaningful insight. Images can also be brought to mind about how you may reduce the pain. For example, if you visualize the pain as hard, red, hot and spiky, you could visualize pouring pure, cold water over the area, making it a blue, cooler colour, softer and more rounded. Another technique is to visualize breathing in a colour to the painful area, which you find soothing and warming, and as you exhale imagine you are breathing away the pain.

Mental transcendence Alternative stimulation, such as music, creative activity, humour, films or other meaningful activities can be used to distract you from or help you to transcend the pain.

Massage As described earlier (see Chapter 3), massage can be extremely helpful in relieving a wide range of cancer-related symptoms, including pain.

Reflexology This therapy is based on the principle that the feet mirror the body and reflex points on the feet correspond to every structure in the body. Like acupuncture it works by balancing energy within the body and also induces relaxation.

Music therapy Music has been shown to alleviate pain in cancer patients. Music can help soothe and calm people; and, used with therapeutic touch and suggestion, it can aid relaxation, improve sleep and decrease anxiety.

Aromatherapy Pain may be caused by a variety of factors and will need specific oils depending on the cause. For best results seek out an aromatherapist. As a general guide, the following oils may be appropriate:

- muscle pain   lavender;
- bone pain   ginger, thyme;
- inflammation   chamomile, eucalyptus, lavender;
- headaches   lavender, lemon;
- stomach cramps   eucalyptus, ginger, peppermint.

The oils may be used in massage, inhalations, oil-burners, aromatic baths or compresses. Always follow the directions for use, and avoid undiluted oil going directly onto your skin.

Cognitive behavioural therapy   This is used to help the person understand if there is a pattern to their pain and to develop appropriate coping mechanisms. The British Association for Behavioural and Cognitive Psychotherapies can help you find a cognitive behavioural therapist; see Appendix 2 for their telephone number.

TENS or TSE   These abbreviations stand for Transcutaneous Electrical Nerve Stimulation or Transcutaneous Spinal Electroanalgesia. A small battery-powered machine sends weak electrical pulses through the skin by means of a pair of rubber pads, which are placed around the painful area or along the spine. This electrical stimulation activates the nerves that block out pain. TENS/TSE can be used throughout the day at regular intervals. Machines can be borrowed from the physiotherapy department at your hospital, or smaller versions may be bought at chemists.

Homoeopathic remedies   Homoeopathy helps to restore health by stimulating the body's natural healing forces. As people vary in their response to illness and there are many different dimensions to pain, homoeopaths prescribe on an individual basis.

Fatigue and Loss of Motivation

Fatigue arises for many reasons, and can be particularly debilitating during and following radiotherapy and chemotherapy. The experience of fatigue under these conditions can be a challenge to relieve. Good nutrition and regular rest, along with gentle regular exercise, have been shown to help fatigue of this nature. In addition to the specific remedies suggested below, massage, self-hypnosis tapes, meditation and visualization can all help to relieve fatigue.

Energy medicines　Acupuncture, homoeopathy, shiatsu, healing and counselling can help access and release emotions that may be causing exhaustion.

Bach Flower Remedies　These help to deal with the underlying emotion:

- olive　　　　　for exhaustion;
- gorse　　　　　for feelings of hopelessness and despair;
- wild rose　　　for resignation and apathy;
- walnut　　　　to assist with change;
- larch　　　　　when confidence is low;
- rock water　　for fear;
- sweet chestnut　for when your thoughts are churning over and over and you are anxious.

Other tips
- Try to set up small, manageable goals each day.
- Take gentle exercise, such as tai chi, yoga, walks; breathe deeply as you walk.
- Try to spend time in nature.
- Accept support; tell your family and friends what you need.
- Allow yourself to feel tired, and to rest.

Nausea
Acupressure　'Sea Bands', which apply pressure on an

acupuncture point on the wrist, are used to prevent or lessen nausea and can be purchased from chemists.

Homoeopathic remedies   As people vary in their response to illness and there are many different causes of nausea, homoeopaths prescribe on an individual basis.

Ginger   Ginger can be used in many forms. To make ginger tea, either use herbal tea bags with ginger or make your own. Simply slice or grate a 1-inch length of ginger (the skin can be left on), pour on boiling water, leave to infuse for five minutes then strain and sweeten with honey if needed.

Alternatively, grate a 2-inch length of ginger with the skin on, gather the grated ginger into your hand and squeeze out the juice. Mix with either water or apple juice. Ginger juice is also good with a mix of carrot and orange juice. Take the ginger tea or juice before and/or after meals and before or during chemotherapy treatment.

Slice a piece of ginger and rub on the pulse points on your wrist when you are feeling nauseous.

Burn ginger essential oil in an oil burner, or simply fill a bowl with boiling water, add one drop of ginger per pint of water, then inhale the steam for five minutes with your eyes closed and a towel over your head if you wish.

Peppermint tea   Peppermint tea bags may be used; or you can make your own with fresh or dried leaves. Inhaling a drop or two of peppermint essential oil on a tissue can provide relief. Do not use peppermint essential oil if you are taking homoeopathic remedies.

Slippery elm   This is the ground inner bark of the slippery elm tree. It is particularly soothing and can bring relief to acidity, oversensitive digestion and nausea. You can find it in most health food stores.

Breathing and relaxation When we feel nauseous we may hold the breath, or breathe in a rapid and shallow manner which may make the nausea worse. By deepening the breath and using relaxation or visualization techniques, we can help relax the body and reduce tension-induced nausea, and also regulate the acid balance in the body if nausea is induced by stress or anxiety.

Bach Flower Remedies These flower essences work not on physical symptoms directly, but on the emotions that surround the ailment. For example, if you feel nauseous due to the fear of chemotherapy, mimulus would be of help, as this is the remedy for a known fear. You can choose the flower remedies yourself; or, for a more holistic and comprehensive assessment of your symptom, it may be wise to consult a practitioner.

Hypnotherapy Hypnotherapists lead clients to contact their subconscious mind, which can help bring about physical or emotional changes. Some people have found this useful for alleviating nausea. Self-hypnosis can also be learned and used to great advantage to cope with stress-induced nausea. For training and guidance in self-hypnosis, make an appointment with a hypnotherapist (see Appendix 2 for contact details).

Prevention Chemotherapy-induced nausea is a side-effect many people experience. However, it is often a psychological response rather than a physical one – although it feels exactly the same whatever its origin! In essence, if you are expecting to feel nauseous from having chemotherapy, it is likely that you will. To combat this, you can practise relaxation, controlled breathing, or visualization techniques which help to view the treatment as a positive experience and reduce anxiety; all these techniques can prevent or very much reduce the feelings of nausea. However, for best effect you will need to establish them in use before you embark on chemotherapy and continue with them throughout the course of treatment.

Breathlessness

Relaxation   Using relaxation techniques on a regular basis, as well as when one is actually suffering with breathlessness, helps the body release the anxiety and stress which can exacerbate this symptom. The body is able to return to a balanced state and the breathing naturally moves into a deeper, slower and more effective rhythm.

Yoga   Yoga works on both body and mind, and so can help alleviate both physical and emotional tension and enhance relaxation. Breathing plays an important part in yoga, which can give you greater awareness and control of your breath.

Breathing techniques   When breathless one often becomes anxious and fearful, and this tends to result in the breath becoming more shallow and rapid. By focusing on the breathing, taking control and using diaphragmatic breathing[61] (see box on pp. 134–5), one can begin to lengthen and deepen the breath, which promotes relaxation and more efficient breathing.

Massage/holding   Massage can be used to release tension in the muscles between the ribs to allow ease of movement when breathing. It can also induce relaxation and well-being, which will have a positive effect on the breath. Simply placing your hands on your abdomen or either side of your chest can be helpful in focusing the mind and helping you to breathe into your hands, which will encourage the breath to deepen and lengthen. You could also get someone else to do this for you.

Digestive Disturbance and Discomfort

Slippery elm   This is the ground inner bark of the slippery elm tree. It is particularly soothing and can bring relief to acidity, diarrhoea, constipation and irritable bowel syndrome. It is also nutritious and soothing, so is excellent in convalescence and if the digestion is weak or oversensitive. You can find it in most health food shops.

Diaphragmatic breathing
Breathing plays a key role in stress and the relaxation response, and as such acts as a link between your mind and body.
Physiologically breathing has two main functions:

- bringing oxygen into the body and sending carbon dioxide out;
- regulating the acid balance in your body.

When you are stressed, anxious or angry, your breathing becomes rapid and shallow and is central to the upper chest area; this is called overbreathing, and leads to poor gaseous exchange in your lungs, resulting in changes to your body chemistry. This imbalance can cause problems such as insomnia, fatigue, reduced energy levels, increased blood cholesterol, high blood pressure and decreased immune function.
You can interrupt persistent overbreathing by diaphragmatic breathing – so called because it pushes the diaphragm, below the lungs, downwards. This brings air to the base of the lungs, thereby improving the efficiency of gaseous exchange, which in turn can induce a relaxation effect and correction of the chemical changes.

Homoeopathic remedies   Ideally, seek out a homoeopath for an individual prescription. Remedies most useful for digestive problems are:

- flatulence and colic   nux vomica;
- food lies like a stone   bryonia;
- bloated after a light meal   lycopodium;
- heartburn   lycopodium;
- aversion to food   ignatia;
- indigestion with flatulence   carbo veg.;
- belching   carbo veg.

Homoeopathic remedies are now widely available in health

Diaphragmatic breathing (continued)
The easiest way to become aware of diaphragmatic breathing
is to place one hand on your chest and one hand on your belly.
As you breathe in, take the air down into your belly: your hand
should rise as your belly expands. Alternatively, you can lie
down and place a book on your belly and watch it rise and fall
with each breath.

It may help to visualize breathing in golden light which
reaches down into your belly; or imagine you have nostrils in
your belly button, and this is the point where you inhale.

It may also help to use positive affirmations as you are
breathing, such as:

- 'I've got all the time in the world to breathe.'
- 'I am going to breathe in / out in a calm manner.'
- 'I have the ability to control how I breathe.'

It takes practice, but you can retrain your diaphragm and
breathing pattern.

The benefits of diaphragmatic breathing are:

- less stress;
- less fatigue;
- improved circulation of blood and lymph flow;
- improved healing;
- a more efficient immune system;
- more positive emotions.

food shops and chemists, and instructions on how best to take
the remedy will be given on the container. Homoeopathy can
also help with loss of appetite.

Peppermint tea   Peppermint tea can be helpful in soothing
and aiding digestion, particularly after eating. Bags may be
used, or you can make your own with fresh or dried leaves. A
drop of peppermint essential oil in some almond oil or baby oil
can be massaged gently on the abdomen. Massage in a clock-

wise direction. Do not use peppermint essential oil if you are taking homoeopathic remedies.

Reflexology   A reflexologist can work on points on the feet that relate to the digestive system to enhance digestion, alleviate constipation and help with loss of appetite.

Acupuncture   Can help with loss of appetite.

Herbal remedies   Many herbal remedies can help with digestion, including loss of appetite; it is best to consult a herbalist or naturopath to guide you to use the most appropriate preparation.

General advice
- Drink plenty of water (aim for 2 litres per day). This will help to replace fluid lost with diarrhoea and to alleviate constipation.
- It often helps to eat small quantities at regular intervals throughout the day, rather than three large meals – especially if weight loss is a problem.
- During chemotherapy, or for people with colostomies, a wholefood diet may be challenging if there are many digestive symptoms. At such times a low residue diet may be helpful. Guidance on this may be obtained from a nutritional therapist.
- If weight loss is a problem, try wholefood build-up drinks (see, for example, the Bristol Centre's recipe in Chapter 6).
- If appetite loss is a problem, try drinking vegetable and fruit juices to boost your nutrient intake.

Minimizing Side-effects

Chemotherapy Side-effects
Nausea   See the above advice on relieving symptoms of nausea; remedies mentioned for appetite loss can help, too. Aloe

vera juice (look for 100% pure juice) can help soothe and heal any damage to the lining of the gastrointestinal tract.

Sore mouth and throat   There are various herbal or homoeopathic mouthwashes which can soothe the mouth; zinc pastilles also provide relief. Colloidal silver (a natural antibiotic) can be used as a mouthwash and then swallowed to provide a systemic effect.

Weakened hair and nails   Hair and nails can be severely affected by chemotherapy. Kelp and other seaweed products can help maintain the condition and strength. Also, massaging almond oil into the nails of both hands and feet increases blood circulation and helps to keep them nourished. The vitamin and mineral programme recommended as part of the Bristol Approach helps with cell regeneration and will, therefore, have an effect on the condition of both hair and nails. Unfortunately, nothing has yet been discovered that will guarantee to prevent hair loss following certain chemotherapy regimes.

Changes to your taste   Sometimes food taste can change during chemotherapy, you may also feel put off by certain foods. This is usually temporary. In our experience, the taste changes that people can experience can vary a great deal from one individual to another. You may find that adding strong flavours to food helps: for example, adding miso paste to soups, or olive paté to sandwiches. Some people, on the other hand, cannot tolerate strong flavours and may find bland soups or the build-up drink (described in Chapter 6) suit them particularly well at this time.

Radiotherapy Side-effects
Digestive disturbance can be a problem for people undergoing radiation therapy; see the section earlier in this chapter (pp. 133–6) for some guidance on ways to minimize this.

A homoeopathic radiation remedy, and Radiance Cream for sore skin (another common side-effect of radiotherapy), are available through the BCHC mail order catalogue.

Bach Flower Remedies Among the appropriate remedies, which act on the emotions surrounding the treatment, are olive (for exhaustion); mimulus (for fear); and crab apple (a cleansing remedy).

Using Relaxation and Visualization to Ease Side-effects

It has been shown that using relaxation techniques, such as muscle relaxation, meditation, visualization, listening to music etc., is associated with less distress, reduction in nausea and lower anxiety following chemotherapy (Walker, 1996; Luebbert, 2001).

Visualization can be used creatively to aid the ability to cope both mentally and physically with chemotherapy. It has been demonstrated to improve nausea symptoms and immune function in breast cancer patients. Carl Simonton's book *Getting Well Again* gives useful instruction in how to use visualization to cope with the experience of chemotherapy.

. . . And After Treatment

- As soon as you are able to, ensure that you are eating as healthily as possible and taking appropriate vitamin and mineral supplements.
- It is important to allow yourself to convalesce. Gently pace yourself back into your usual daily routines. Assess what your usual routines were before treatment, and take the chance to review your priorities.
- Look at Chapter 6 on 'life review' to start to reflect on your needs. Consider its suggestions on how to move forward and look ahead after diagnosis and treatment.

A visualization to support you through radiotherapy
Before and after radiotherapy, try the following visualization:

Relax the body using the breath as a focus, extending the exhalation and letting go on the exhalation, continue for a few breaths using the breath to calm and centre yourself. Picture the rays being immensely beneficial – helping to destroy the cancer, and only the cancer cells. See the tumour shrinking and disappearing, protective light filling all the healthy cells around the tumour. Picture yourself radiantly well and at peace.

6

Life Review:
Getting Yourself Going

This chapter is designed to help you look ahead and plan your life following initial diagnosis and treatment. It first looks in turn at all the areas of your life that can affect your health and suggests how you might arrange them to bring maximum benefit to yourself. It concludes with guidance on setting therapeutic priorities, learning to take care of yourself, and pacing the changes you may decide to bring about in your life.

Moving On After Diagnosis and Treatment

Faced with the shock of a cancer diagnosis, and then with the challenge of treatment, it is difficult immediately to set about reviewing your lifestyle. Following treatment, however, you may wish to reflect and explore how you can now move forward in the most creative way possible for you in your own particular personal circumstances. This is what this chapter sets out to help you to do.

The chapter contains a variety of exercises that you can do, and also opportunities for reflection. You may wish to buy a special notebook, in which you will enjoy writing, where you can capture these reflections.

Whether it is through embarking upon the Bristol Approach, or by making your own assessment of your state and needs, it is important to determine your therapeutic priorities and to decide which therapies you will use. You will then need to know how to go about finding the best therapists in your area to give you the help you need. (See box at end of Chapter 3 for guidance on choosing a complementary therapist.)

In this chapter we shall concentrate on the primary factors that affect your overall health, and the ways in which you can begin to control them. Though of course they are interlinked, for the ease of exploration it seems best to break them down and consider them one by one.

There are seven main areas that you will need to look at and assess:

- your spiritual state;
- your energy levels;
- your emotional and mental state;
- your physical state;
- your environment;
- your lifestyle;
- your relationships.

Spiritual State

The most important factor – of fundamental importance to your overall health and well-being – is the state of your spirit. To assess your spiritual state, you will need to begin by asking yourself two vital questions:

- Do I really have the will to live?

- Does my life still have a purpose and meaning that is genuinely to do with me and my own self-expression (rather than with being here purely for others, be they children, elderly parents or partner)?

Of course, the other people in your life are vital considerations; but it is really important to look at how your unique life energy is expressed. This leads into the question whether or not you have sources of uplift and nourishment for your spirit, and whether you take the time to build these into your life – and behind all of this is the question of whether you feel fundamentally connected to life and society, or whether you have come to feel isolated and separate.

If you recognize that your spirit is crushed, or that you feel disillusioned or lost in life, it would be extremely beneficial to get involved either in the Bristol Approach or in transpersonal psychotherapy to literally 'bring yourself back to life'. It may also be important to have spiritual healing regularly to lift your spirit.

Laurence LeShan, one of the grandfathers of holistic medicine, had a very strong sense that sometimes people became ill when they lost touch with themselves and their passion for living. He suggested various exercises to help people reconnect with the style of life that allows for enthusiasm and involvement – a reconnection that can in fact make life far better after the illness than it was before.

If this sounds like an important message for you, try this two-part exercise, which may help you reconnect with your true purpose in life.

Exercise: What Makes Your Heart Sing?
First, try to write down some answers to the following questions.

What activities make you feel more alive and vital? (If you find this difficult, take a moment to record joyous times in your life and see what they have in common.)

What activities seem to drain me?   (Recall when you have felt your energy levels diminish, and what seems to precede this feeling.)

Is there a balance in my life between work and play?   (To help you here, try to write down three or four things you do as 'work' and the same number for 'play'.)

Now, reading and reflecting on what you have written, think what changes you can make in your life in the next week / month / year to be living your life with as much zest, enthusiasm and passion as possible.

The next week

The next month

The next year

Energy Levels

Assessing Your Energy State

At the beginning of any holistic health programme – and indeed, from then onwards on a day-to-day basis – it is extremely important to ask yourself what is going on with your energy.

To start getting a real sense of your own energy state, you need to try to 'tune in' to what is happening to your energy. This is easiest to do after a relaxation exercise. Often people will say, 'My energy levels are great – I can keep going for hours and hours,' but the minute they relax and let go they discover that they are too exhausted to stay awake. This phenomenon occurs when people override the body's signals of exhaustion by 'pumping themselves up', often with the aid of coffee, cigarettes and other stimulants; this way, they induce the feeling of 'high energy' although in fact they are actually running on empty. It is continuing to work hard for prolonged periods in this kind of state that often results in 'burn-out' or the 'TATT [tired all the time] syndrome': burn-out occurs when the override mechanism finally breaks down and the individual is forced to acknowledge the depth of his or her tiredness.

Apportioning Your Energy Appropriately

The next step has two parts.

First you must analyse where or how you are expending all your energy, and whether it is in ways that really profit you or that leave you unsatisfied, resentful or even feeling abused. Review the section of Chapter 2 on 'Energy and Life Force' – especially the exercise where you gave yourself 100 points to represent all the energy you had in a typical week and apportioned it among the categories of your life to see where it went. Consider again:

- whether you spend most of your energy in one area, and
- how much you put aside for yourself.

Then you must identify the things that refresh you and genuinely give you energy. Once you have made these distinctions, you can begin to replace the former with the latter.

As you become better at staying in touch with your energy state, you can get down to finer and finer tuning as you begin to ask yourself: 'Do I really wish to put my energy into that phone call, that shopping trip into the centre of town, organizing that event, propping up that draining relationship? Or do I wish to let these things go so that I can conserve and build my energy and enjoy using it?'

You may also begin to notice how much of your energy is wasted through accumulation of physical tension in the body, or by 'over-egging the pudding' socially or professionally. Do you put twice as much energy into everything as you really need to, and feel resentful when others don't notice or don't appreciate all the effort you have made?

A Word of Caution: Low Energy Levels

If, when making your initial assessment of your energy state, you realize that your energy levels are very low, then it is important to pull back immediately from your normal commitments and to start seeing a healer or a practitioner of acupuncture, shiatsu or homoeopathy, so that you can begin to build your vital energy again quickly.

Start one step at a time; do not exhaust your energies by trying to tackle too many things at once. If you are still unsure where to start with your programme for self-healing, look at the 'inner reflections' exercise at the end of this chapter (pp. 168–70).

Emotional and Mental State

You will need to assess your emotional and mental state both in terms of your reaction to diagnosis and treatment of cancer, and in terms of the state that predominated prior to diagnosis.

The beginning of Chapter 3 went into some detail about the effects of the shock of diagnosis. It is very likely that in the short term you will need a counsellor to help you express the distress you are feeling, grieve for the losses you are experiencing, and gradually enable you to get your feet back on the ground, somewhat adjusted to the reality of the situation you are now facing. Some people prefer to do this in a support group with others going through the same experience. It can be extremely helpful to meet other people who are living with cancer, because they will understand exactly how you feel.

While your tendency may be to 'batten down the hatches' or 'get a grip', it is far better for you to try to let go at this point. This applies to your family and other close relationships as well as to the counselling or support group context. The combination of the fear levels you may be experiencing and the effort of 'being nice' or 'striving for harmony' can be exhausting and make it difficult to sustain solid, intimate relationships. It is very possible that you may be able to use this time of heightened intensity to choose to abandon these strategies or ways of being, and reorientate yourself around new motivations and core values associated with your personal fulfilment and creative self-expression.

Within the field of cancer medicine, and the support services that surround it, there is increasing provision for help in the initial distress that accompanies diagnosis, either through access to specialist nurse counsellors, or through counselling provided routinely by your oncology unit or GP's practice. One of the benefits of the transpersonal counselling approach used at Bristol is that it enables people with cancer and their supporters to look very deeply at how their normal state of mind and emotional reality is affecting their body's ability to resist or recover from disease.

If you wish to embark on this kind of self-examination, or have a sense that your established way of relating emotionally is putting strain on you, then the courses at the Bristol Cancer Help Centre will be highly appropriate, as will finding a transpersonal counsellor in your own area to continue the counselling process locally (or to initiate such counselling if you are unable to come to Bristol). Unlike psychoanalysis, transpersonal counselling is not usually a long process. You may find that your psychological reorientation occurs within only weeks of having regular sessions. (For a description of transpersonal counselling, look back at Chapter 3, pp. 61–6.)

Exercise: All About You

Here is a reflection exercise from the Bristol Cancer Help Centre's art therapist, Diana Brueton, which uses the creative medium of art to explore how you see yourself at the moment, what you are wanting in your life and how you might achieve it.

You'll need four sheets of paper and something to draw or paint with.

1   Quickly think of a shape or symbol which represents how you are feeling right now, and draw it on the first sheet of paper. For example:

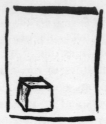

2   On the second piece of paper, draw a shape or symbol that stands for how you would *like* to be. Again, work as spontaneously as possible. For example:

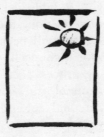

3   On the next sheet, draw both the previous shapes, for example:

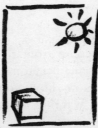

Make sure you position the drawings on the paper as they were originally. Are they a long way apart, close or even superimposed? Does the space that separates them have meaning to you?

4 Now think about how you might bring these two shapes together – in other words, what things might help you to move towards the 'you' of the second drawing. On your fourth sheet, repeat the drawing you just did, but now add in connections between the two shapes, using whatever shapes, patterns, symbols you like. For instance:

Feel that these connections are now starting to happen: you are creating them.

This is a great exercise to do whenever you are feeling unsure of how to move forward.

Facing the Fears

An extremely important part of the holistic approach is learning to look absolutely head-on at the things that are scaring you. Of course, you need the right level of support and 'holding' in order to do this. This may come from an individual counsellor or from a group. It is quite remarkable how much better you will feel if you can allow yourself to name and explore your fears.

Finding the real fear When you begin to do this, you will quite probably discover that the thing that is really worrying you is not quite what you thought it was. For example, people who say they are terrified of operations quite often find that it is not the operation itself that scares them but rather the implicit loss of control. When they find out exactly what it is that is bothering them, it becomes possible to start doing something about it – for example, in this case, conveying the fear to healthcare professionals; asking them to give you as much information as humanly possible about what is going to happen and how you will get help if you need it; what procedures, tubes and stitches you will have; how you will get pain relief; whether you can give the final go-ahead to the anaesthetist when you feel ready; and so on.

Similarly, when people examine their fear of dying, they often discover that it is not so much dying itself that frightens them but rather the question of how they will die: whether they will suffer, whether they will be 'a nuisance to others', whether the process will involve their becoming disabled and dependent – losing control – and having to allow others, who don't know them that well, to take over at such a significant time, when they feel at their most vulnerable. Often the greatest fear of all is the pain of letting go of relatives and loved ones. But in 'speaking the unspeakable', and by grieving and 'finishing the emotional business' with others, immense relief can be found. And in being helped to think about, or even plan, your dying process – however far in the future it may be – and talking about this to your closest carers, you can also be relieved of a great deal of worry and stress.

Sharing the fear   Once you have tackled these really big fears – and realized how much better you feel when you can look at and communicate what is going on inside – you may find that you get a taste for it. This means that you can look at what is frightening you regularly, first with your counsellor but later perhaps with others with whom you have personal relationships. You can take turns with your loved ones to say what you are feeling, and then what you need. For the other person, the object is not to intervene or necessarily even say anything; rather, it is to provide a supportive listening presence, while resisting the urge to find solutions or 'make you feel better'. For you, the object of expressing your feelings is not to prompt the other person to jump in and try to fulfil a need, but rather to bring them to full consciousness, which not only makes you feel better but means that you have a much clearer map of what is going on for you. Quite often you will find that the process of articulating these things changes them, and begins to alter the way you feel, liberating you to move on through and out of the other side of this dark forest of fears.

Physical State

When starting to assess your physical state, the main questions you will need to ask yourself are:

- How do I eat?
- What is my body's state of fitness?
- How do I hold myself posturally, and what are my breathing patterns like?
- Am I holding a lot of stress and tension in my body?
- How well do I express my physicality in dance and sport?

Diet

If your eating is far from healthy, you may need the help of a nutritional therapist to guide you into a healthy eating pattern and to give you the emotional support necessary to make the changes. Changing the way we eat can be difficult, especially if there are other stresses in our lives; it is very important to do it in a way that will minimize the risk of failure, and a nutritional therapist will help you do this.

Sample meals with which to construct your menus

Breakfast
- Organic muesli, possibly soaked overnight with soya milk, oat milk, rice milk or juice, rice or oat porridge
- Fresh fruit salad or stewed fruit compote
- Wholemeal toast with soya margarine, honey or sugar-free jam with sweeteners
- Herb tea or vegetable/fruit juice
- An occasional organic free-range boiled egg with wholemeal toast

Mid-morning
- Fruit, vegetable or fruit juice; snack of homemade flapjack, or nuts and seeds

Lunch
- Fresh salad with mixed leaves, sprouts, grated or chopped vegetables, nuts, seeds, dried fruits, or cooked beans with home-made salad dressing
- Home-made vegetable soup, fortified with barley or rice if desired
- Wholefood pie or pasty
- Organic wholemeal brown bread with hummus, avocado, nut butters or vegetable paté
- Mixed salad using grains such as pasta, rice, buckwheat, quinoa
- Fresh fruit

Because the subject of healthy eating is such a big one, the Bristol Cancer Help Centre's Head Chef and Dietary Adviser, Jane Sen, has written two *Healing Foods* cookbooks explaining the principles and setting out a wide range of recipes and techniques. These will help you to prepare and use nutritious foods in an exciting and appetizing way. Details of the books, and three videos on food and drink preparation techniques, are given in Appendix 1.

Sample meals (continued)

Mid-afternoon
- Fruit, vegetable or fruit juice; snack of homemade flapjack, or nuts and seeds

Dinner
- Mixed vegetables with a little steamed wild fish or organic chicken
- Mixed-leaf salad with home-made vinaigrette
- Vegetarian lentil shepherd's pie with steamed mixed vegetables
- Baked bananas with cinnamon-date syrup, with soya cream, soya ice cream or soya yoghurt
- Fruit jelly (using agar flakes)
- Herb tea or coffee substitute

Water should be sipped freely throughout the day.

The main emphasis in the Centre's dietary guidelines is on increasing the amount of (preferably organic) vegetables and fruits in your diet while simultaneously reducing the amount of animal fat, meat, salt, sugary foods and processed foods to an absolute minimum. Some typical meals from which to construct your daily menus are shown in the boxes on these pages. In principle, healthy eating will involve rebuilding your diet around wholefoods: pulses, nuts, seeds and the many different grains. This can be very exciting and, with the help of Jane Sen, either directly or through reading her books, it can become a really creative pleasure, and you will discover how delicious this food can be.

One of the top tips for avoiding failure when changing your diet is to start by including more of the good things before getting rid of those that are not good for you. For instance, you can first include vegetables or fruit in every meal; you can then

Build-up drink
This recipe is a very tasty and easy-to-make high-protein, high-calorie, dairy-free drink. It is particularly helpful to take this if you are trying to increase your weight. If you do not have a very big appetite, take it in between meals; it should not be used as a meal replacement except on occasions when you really do not fancy anything else.

4 oz plain tofu (organic fresh or silken)
1 pt soya milk
1 banana
1 tbsp organic maple syrup
1 tbsp slippery elm powder
1/2 tsp vanilla essence

Blend all ingredients together in liquidizer until smooth.

Possible additions and variations
2 tbsp ground almonds
2 tbsp cooked brown rice (or cooked whole grains, e.g. millet or oats)
Any fresh fruit
2 tbsp cooked dried fruits (apricots are lovely)
A little honey or concentrated apple juice
1 or 2 drops of almond essence
1 tbsp organic, sugar-free fruit preservative

begin to replace everything that is white with the brown equivalent, e.g. bread, rice, pasta and flour; and then you can begin to substitute vegetarian products for their animal counterparts – particularly butter, cheese, meat, cream and milk.

If you feel protein-hungry and are not satisfied by vegetarian proteins, eat some deep-sea fish (or fish that has not been farmed), have two to three eggs a week, and occasionally have some organic free-range meat (preferably chicken or game).

It is also wise to drink plenty of high-quality water (around 2 litres or 4 pints per day). If you like, this can taken as herbal tea.

Ten top nutrition tips
- Cook brown rice in bulk, then cool quickly and rinse thoroughly under the cold tap and freeze in portions. To use, add rice to boiling water for 5 minutes, strain and serve.
- Put a mixture of seeds – sunflower, pumpkin, linseed and sesame – in a clean pepper mill and grind onto meals.
- Carry a 2-litre bottle of water around with you, or put it on your desk, and make sure you drink it by the end of the day.
- Try one new vegan recipe each week to build up your repertoire.
- Carry some fruit with you for a quick pick-me-up.
- Always have a small pack of dried fruit, nuts and seeds with you, so that you have a ready snack and aren't tempted to buy junk food.
- A few salad leaves at the beginning of a meal helps digestion.
- Leave three hours between finishing your evening meal and going to bed.
- Do a menu plan for a whole week so that you know what you are going to cook each night – it saves lots of time!
- When you prepare a healthy meal, make twice as much as you need and freeze half of it for another day.

Between meals – mid-morning, teatime and mid-evening – it is also good to make yourself fresh vegetable or fruit juice. To do this you will need to invest in a juice extractor, which can be obtained from electrical suppliers. The most basic models are centrifugal, which are adequate for the purpose. At the other end of the spectrum you will find juice-presses, which are thought to be less destructive of the plant enzymes but are about ten times the price of the centrifugal juicers.

Supplementing your diet with a vitamin and mineral schedule is also important (see Chapter 3).

Your vitamins can be obtained by mail order or by phone from Can Help Now, the Bristol Cancer Help Centre's trading company (see Appendix 1). This method of obtaining your vitamins is easy and efficient, and there is the added advantage of knowing that you are benefiting the Centre's charity. Fine-tuning of your vitamin recommendations, and suggestions about other metabolic support, will be given by your doctor at the Centre or elsewhere.

Stress, Tension and Relaxation

Very often when people consider their physical state after a diagnosis of cancer they focus solely on the part of their body that is directly affected by the cancer. It is important to remember that the whole of you needs to be maintained in as strong and healthy a state as possible. At a time of heightened emotion the body is likely to be expressing this as physical tension somewhere within your body. You may know for yourself your 'weak spots' – perhaps a tendency at stressful times to get headaches, backache, a stiff neck or shoulders. It will therefore be important for you to reflect on what is the most effective way for you to release the tension. For some people bodywork may be helpful; for others the best way is to relax the mind, either by talking your problems through with a counsellor or learning techniques such as relaxation and meditation to help quieten the mind. A combination of both approaches would be ideal. If you are finding it a real challenge to accept your diagnosis and resist the emotions that have arisen since it was presented to you, or if you feel you are in a state of heightened anxiety and your mind is very busy, counselling may be particularly helpful.

You may find that bodywork or relaxation therapies help in the short term but your mind continually disrupts the peace; in that case, it may be more appropriate for you to start by settling the mind. Other people find that trying bodywork or relaxation therapies first quietens the mind and the body then softens and releases the tension, opening up the way back to health and restoration. You will need to find the best way for you at this time, your own unique way of dealing with your situation.

Exercise and Physical Expression

All of us require exercise. We should take at least 20 minutes of aerobic exercise twice a week. But this may simply not be realistic for you at present, in which case a stretching routine may be more appropriate. We all need to stretch (as cats and dogs demonstrate so beautifully). Many of us have very sedentary lifestyles, spending hours in front of desks, driving cars, or sitting in front of TVs or computers. It is important to stretch our spines, joints, muscles, ligaments and tendons; this has the effect of 'massaging' our internal organs, which ensures that the blood flow to all areas of the body remains good; this in turn helps to prevent the build-up of toxicity or calcium deposits in the tissues where cancer tends to develop. So, whatever happens, a basic stretch and breathe routine, such as the one taught on the Bristol therapy programme, will serve you very well in your recovery process. It would also be extremely helpful to seek out local yoga, tai chi or chi gong classes.

You may be the sort of person for whom physical expression is an important part of your creativity, but have abandoned this part of yourself as the pressures of parenthood or work mounted, or as inertia took over. If you know deep down that your body aches to dance, jump, climb, hang-glide, skate or run, then it is extremely important that you should respond to this and start doing it (though you should of course break yourself in again gently). Cancer rates are considerably lower in people who exercise, and it may be very significant that Penny Brohn, who lived for 20 years with breast cancer and its bony recurrences, swam 50 lengths three times a week until very near the end of her life.

Exercise: stretching   Try if you can to start each day with a stretching session. Before undertaking any stretching exercise please check with your doctor – especially if you have a history of bone cancer, osteoporosis or arthritis.

- Stand with your feet hip-width apart and stretch your arms up, first one side then the other, pointing the toe on the opposite side simultaneously.

- Then rotate your shoulders in their joints to loosen the shoulder muscles. Gently rotate your neck, applying a little lift to the head as you do so in order that you do not stress the vertebrae in the neck. (The head is a lot heavier than you think.)

- Next put the feet about 1 metre (40 inches) apart; allow yourself to bend forward, and put your hands on the floor. If it is comfortable, place one hand in the central position and then, twisting your spine, lift the other arm above your head, and look upwards. Repeat on the other side. Be gentle with yourself – do not go past your comfortable limit.

- From this position go onto all fours, and then stretch the spine like a cat, first of all upwards – tucking your chin into your chest – and then dipping or hollowing your back and extending your head and neck upwards and backwards. Once you have the hang of this, give some attention to your breathing at the same time: inhale as you hollow your spine, and exhale as you arch your back upwards. Repeat this process very slowly and smoothly, and really enjoy the feeling.

- Then, if you are able, come to a sitting position on the floor, and gently bend forward into your maximum stretch position without any pushing or pulling or straining of the muscles.

- Uncurl gently, and lie flat on the floor on your back for a few minutes so that you can absorb the benefits of these stretches.

A basic day plan
A good structure for your daily programme would be:

Morning

7.00–7.15	Glass of hot or cold water with lemon before stretching
7.15–7.45	Relaxation and meditation
8.00–9.00	Wholefood breakfast plus vitamins and mineral supplements
11.00	Freshly made vegetable juice with wholefood biscuits and fruit

Afternoon

1.00	Wholefood lunch, plus vitamins and minerals
4.00	Freshly made juice, with wholefood cake or biscuits or fruit

Evening

7.00–8.00	Wholefood dinner, plus vitamins and minerals
9.00–9.30	Meditation
9.30	Rice cakes, oatcakes, almonds
10.00	Zinc tablet. Relaxing bath with candles and oils; bedtime

Just these simple stretches will invigorate you no end, making it much easier to do all your other self-help activities.

In addition to this stretching routine, try to include a walk or swim, and opportunities for plenty of fresh air, as part of your weekly routine. Ideally, once you are able, add a regular visit to a yoga, tai chi or chi gong class.

You will soon experience great benefits from increasing your physical activity. Over time, your energy levels will increase so much that you will find your need for therapy will drop away. At this stage you will be strong enough to motivate yourself to maintain this self-help activity, and will go from strength to strength.

Use of Bodywork

Consider regular massage or shiatsu sessions as part of your ongoing support programme. These can help with continuing symptoms, such as scars, lymphoedema, insomnia and so forth, as described in Chapter 3. Regular bodywork can boost your energy levels and also your self-esteem at times of challenge or difficulty.

Bodywork can also provide much-needed relaxation and physical pleasure. This can be most valuable in rebuilding and maintaining intimate relationships – if you feel good about your body, you are more likely to experience yourself as a sexual being.

Sexuality

It may be important to ask how your sexual energy is manifesting itself, as unexpressed sexual energy may make us bad tempered or violent, obsessive or driven.

The issue of how to express our sexuality fully is a complex one, because much depends on our compatibility with – or, indeed, the presence of – a partner. If, for whatever reason, we feel 'stuck' or limited in our sexuality, help is available either conventionally, from sex therapists, or through Tantra training. Tantra is a form of yoga in which one learns how to channel sexual energy into the higher energy centres or chakras in the body in order to open ourselves to higher states of consciousness. It can be very helpful as it provides an alternative, but satisfactory and enjoyable, way of expressing this energy.

The Tantra training offered in Britain currently focuses on what it is that gets in the way of our pleasure and enjoyment of our sexuality, and how we can heal the shame, inhibition, fear and abusive elements of our sexuality. This fits in very well with the holistic approach. Both couples and single people can undertake and benefit from Tantra training.

Environment

Health problems can be caused by environmental stresses, either social or physical. For example, many people have helped themselves to become well by removing themselves from the influence of a very overpowering personal relationship – 'taking back their power' – and re-establishing their autonomy. Similarly, people have become well again after recognizing that the building, or even the city, in which they live or work, makes them feel unwell. Your home environment can be checked for what is called geopathic stress; this is done by dowsers or physicists, who look for high and low areas of magnetic, electromagnetic or radioactive energy, which can markedly affect health.

The main thing is to trust your intuition. If you quieten down, perhaps with the help of relaxation, meditation and visualization, and ask yourself how your living and working environment is making you feel, you may well be surprised to discover how much you already know and the extent to which you have been ignoring your own 'inner knowing'.

Lifestyle

Assessing Lifestyle Balance
Your lifestyle will reflect the state of your spirit, emotions and mind, and vice versa. Ask yourself these questions:

- Am I balancing my work with leisure activities, my times of busyness with stillness?
- Do I take time purely for myself, without planned activity, to be reflective and develop creativity?

If, in answering these questions, you can see that your lifestyle is out of balance and that your quality of living has become severely reduced, it can be useful, with the help of a holistic doctor or counsellor, to address this problem head-on and decide how you are going to make the appropriate changes.

Letting Go and Making Space

This will inevitably mean some letting go. Many of us are workaholic or perfectionist, or perhaps just plain greedy in terms of the amount we take on. We can't bear to abandon our projects or hand them over to others with whom they may fail – or, worse still, do better than when we were at the helm! Some of us are so bad at controlling our work that we allow it to leak into and take over all areas of our life; in such cases we need to schedule time with ourselves and our families, or put our new creative or self-help activity into the diary in the same way we would timetable work appointments. This can be a good trick in establishing a new lifestyle – entering these times into the diary a long way ahead, and fitting work activity around them as opposed to the other way around.

Some of us require a physical symbol of this space for ourselves in our lives. This might take the form of a room of our own, or even an area in an existing room in the house, where we can be 'in our own space', surrounded by what is significant to us. Usually it is people whose lives are the most caught up in the needs of others who most strongly need to take this action.

Relationships

Your Relationships with Yourself and Others

Almost everything that has been mentioned so far in this chapter is about developing a new relationship with yourself. The very process of asking yourself questions and evaluating your state means that you have begun to take notice of how you are and how the things around you affect you. It is important to think clearly about what time, attention and care you give yourself, and what this says about your relationship with yourself. Ask yourself whether you think you are actually abusive towards yourself. For instance:

- Do I harm myself with cigarettes or excessive alcohol or drugs?
- Do I set myself crazy targets or actually harm myself physically?
- Do I stay in relationships in which I am being hurt or mistreated?

You may be prone to chronically abandoning yourself – that is, putting everybody else's needs before your own. Further, you may despise yourself for getting caught up in sadomasochistic relationships with yourself and others, and this can initiate and maintain a cycle of allowing yourself to be abused. These cyclical patterns can take myriad different forms and involve any number of different people – parents, colleagues, lovers and friends – but whatever the context, the effect is to leave you feeling alienated and unnourished.

The dynamics of our relationship with ourselves will determine how much love we are able to let in, how much help we will allow ourselves to receive, and whether we will be able to build a new life that is balanced, wholesome and healthy, and truly reflects who we are.

Honesty with ourselves is the key to finding out what we need to do. If we know that in our relationships with others we have been habitually rather dominant, overpowering and selfish, we may need to learn how to soften, to listen, and to serve the needs of others. If our pattern has been to abandon ourselves and allow ourselves to be dominated, we shall need to learn how to know and express our needs, and to become more assertive.

How successful we are in breaking these cycles in relationships with others will ultimately depend on whether we can bear to be on our own until a new, healthier relationship develops. This in turn depends on our developing a new relationship with ourselves: as we become less needy and dependent, we compromise ourselves less and become more self-sufficient.

There are many ways we can develop better relationships with ourselves and others, either through help from a skilled counsellor or through developmental group work.

Your Relationship with Life and the Divine
Ask yourself the following questions:

- Do I feel supported by life, or do I feel like an island, permanently cut off and battling for survival?
- Do I believe in the possibility that there is a planetary life force or higher, intelligent, loving consciousness that can assist me, or do I, on the contrary, feel entirely separate and alone in the world?

Two of the most powerful experiences people have in embracing the holistic approach are, first, the discovery of their own personal power, which becomes apparent as they begin to develop both their sense of purpose and their creative will through visualization and affirmation processes (of which more in Chapter 7), and, second, the discovery of how much loving help there is within the universe if they only become receptive to it and ask for it.

To make the first discovery involves moving out of a passive relationship with life and beginning, through the processes of visualization and affirmation, to start choosing the way you want things to be. This can be done in images or in words, and is remarkably powerful. Practising visualization brings one up against one's 'limiting beliefs', which are the voices that tell us we can't possibly be successful or have things the way we want them. Given sufficient encouragement and support, however, these barriers can be crossed, with very exciting results. But equally exciting is the diametrically opposite process, which is learning to 'let go and let God'. For people who constantly take control in all situations, this moment may be reached only in extremis. For others, beginning the process of 'handing over to a higher power' comes more easily.

Just as taking control of your own life sets free a whole set of forces that can then come to your assistance, so letting go and surrendering to God or the universe, and asking for the appropriate help, can set in motion another set of processes that allows all manner of unforeseen help to come to your assistance and to the assistance of those around you. Formal help is available to assist you in initiating these processes, but both are much simpler than you may imagine at first.

These two processes can be seen as forming an apparently paradoxical but highly effective blueprint for living for all of us – directing us towards being able to move back and forth between our active, creative, individuated self, and our surrendered, expanded sense of self, where we give up our sense of control and hand over our trust to the life process. In establishing this level of flexibility we can develop a very strong sense of self while simultaneously learning to let go and 'go with the flow' of life, even if ultimately this means flowing into our dying. As one spiritual teacher said, 'We must learn how to take hold tightly and let go lightly.'

Therapeutic Priorities

Reading through this section on the holistic life appraisal will have given you an idea of what is going through the minds of doctors, counsellors, healers, nurses and therapists at the Bristol Cancer Help Centre as they take you through the therapeutic assessment processes. Once your needs are established, you and your therapy team can determine your therapeutic priorities. These may include help in facing the cancer diagnosis, making treatment decisions, going through and coping with cancer treatments and dealing with the symptoms of your illness, and the much bigger process of setting about promoting your health 'from the inside out'.

Your therapeutic priorities will change over time as healing begins to take place, and this is why regular reassessment and review are important.

Learning to Care for Yourself

If you have never really thought much about yourself or your needs, perhaps the biggest challenge of all when adopting the holistic approach is that of learning to care for yourself. One visitor to the Centre recalled a comment made by one of her therapists at home: 'Think carefully about getting involved with the holistic approach – it will involve your committing yourself, your time and your money to the process.' The person involved had at first recoiled, thinking, 'I can't possibly do that – spend money on, and take time for, myself – how selfish.' But, as the days went on, she gradually realized that investing in herself was the essence of the holistic recovery process.

In order to help people become accustomed to the idea of forging this new relationship with themselves, we suggest that they think of themselves as a child in their own care. If this child were ill they would make absolutely sure the child went to bed early, had lots of treats and words of encouragement, and the best and most nourishing food; if the child had no appetite, they would sit with them at mealtimes and try all manner of means to tempt them to eat.

For some people, establishing this new relationship with the self can be quite daunting, and they find it difficult to know where to start. In such cases it helps to begin the process gradually: make a few simple changes that are sustainable, and then begin to take further steps towards bigger changes as the needs become apparent. Other people see absolutely clearly the

Caring for yourself – the essential ingredients

- Think about *getting it right for yourself* in all situations. While this may initially feel selfish and uncomfortable – like crossing your arms the wrong way – you will quickly find that if you learn to get things right for you it will be far better for everybody else around you.
- *Take time for yourself.* Allocate several days and evenings a month which are solely your time. Make this unstructured time that you can use as appropriate when it arrives. Use these times to be reflective, and to do only things that soothe, nurture and lift your spirit. In addition to this, make regular time for your important therapeutic sessions or self-help classes.
- *Be gentle with yourself.* Do not make the holistic approach another stick with which to beat your back. There are absolutely no shoulds or oughts involved in any of the many aspects of the holistic approach. It is not about setting yourself gigantic tasks, feeling guilty if you fail, and in general assuming too great a responsibility for yourself and your health. Quite the reverse: it is about identifying the aspects of yourself that tend to push you too hard, and allowing yourself to find a new way of being – one that is gentle, spontaneous and feels very right to you. Remember, you are the only one who can judge that.
- *Prioritize* activities that excite and enthuse you, and allow you self-expression.
- *Let go* of your concerns about the opinions of others.
- Most important of all, *be yourself*.

changes they need to make from early on in the process of self-appraisal, and they may be able to make dramatic changes in one fell swoop. In all cases, the healing journey is intensely personal, and should be undertaken at your own pace. It is very important not to judge yourself or compare yourself with others who may appear to be doing more than you. Often the inner changes people make can have more profound effects than the dramatic-looking external life changes.

Inner Reflection

One of the problems with a holistic approach to healing is that it is sometimes a bit difficult to know where to begin. If you are lucky you will have an inclination towards a particular source of healing. You may have heard a bit about using diet as therapy, which would make nutrition the obvious place to start; or you may have caught on to the idea that cancer is stress-related, and look around for a counsellor.

If you don't know where to start, here is an exercise that has been well used at the Bristol Cancer Help Centre since our co-founder Penny Brohn was involved to help people reflect on their needs.

Exercise: Inner Reflections

Give yourself half an hour free of interruptions and obligations.

Find four chairs and put them in a square, facing inwards, so that each is facing one other. On the floor in front of each chair put a piece of paper on which you have identified each chair with a part of yourself:

1 your higher self, your spirit;
2 your physical body;
3 your rational, logical, thinking self;
4 your emotional, feeling self.

You should not have much difficulty in seeing a distinction between your physical body and your mental activity, but some people have to work at seeing a difference between their rational, intelligent self and their emotional, intuitive self. There are an awful lot of people who say 'I feel' when they really mean 'I think'! You might mull over that for a minute or two.

If you are uneasy about the word 'spirit', see how you feel with 'soul' or 'collective unconscious'. The idea is to find a word for that part of you that is not physical/mechanical or emotional/logical, but that is detached from all these processes. The part of you that is your own 'wise observer'. You could even call it that.

1   Start in the chair labelled Higher Self, Spirit or whatever. Relax and close your eyes. Think about the idea that there is a part of you that is watching the rest of you, that is not tangled up with your comings or goings; a part that is detached and free. Allow yourself to feel refreshed by this idea. Try to let go of all the other aspects of yourself and have an awareness of this wise companion that you have with you all the time.

If any special thoughts or symbols come into your head, write them down on the piece of paper.

2   Move into the chair labelled Physical Body. Relax and close your eyes. Wander around your body. Which parts of you do you like or dislike? Are you hungry? Are you cold? How does your body feel about the way you look after it?

If any special thoughts or symbols come into your head, write them down on the paper.

Return for a moment or two to the chair for your Higher Self.

3   Move to the chair labelled Logical, Rational Self. What's going on here? Is your intellect being exercised in the life you lead? Are you listening to your own wisdom? What do you know and understand, as distinct from what you sense and feel?

If any special thoughts and symbols come into your head, write them down on the paper.

Go back for a few moments and get in touch again with your Higher Self.

4   Sit in the chair that is labelled Emotions and Feelings. What are your emotions right now? What are you feeling? Are there certain emotions you feel comfortable with and others you

avoid? Do you want to cry? To laugh? To shout?

If any special thoughts or symbols come into your head, write them down on the paper.

Return for a final few moments with your Higher Self.

You can take the chairs in any order you like, but after each one return for a minute or two to the Higher Self. This means that while you will occupy the chairs for the body, the mind and the emotions just once each, you will occupy the one representing your Higher Self four times in all.

In time you will find it useful to address a specific question to the various aspects of yourself, but to begin with just try to identify clearly with the different parts and find out what's going on with each of them. See what they have to say to you.

This is a very simple exercise that you can do on your own and you can repeat it whenever you like. Always keep the pieces of paper, even if they are all blank! Date them and toss them in a box. You won't be sorry, because they will make a fascinating record. Pay special attention to any images or symbols that come up and note them in your book. Later you may be able to incorporate them into affirmations or visualizations.

Making Progress

You will soon find that reviewing your life systematically in the way described in this chapter, and setting about reorganizing and prioritizing with your own true needs in view – if possible with regular therapeutic input from your healer, counsellor and/or energy therapist – will make a very big difference to your state and ability to cope. You may even start to glimpse the potential that is involved in this crisis.

As noted earlier in this book, in Chapter 2, working with the holistic approach can be compared to renovating a garden. Think of yourself as both garden and gardener, and set about the renovation process in stages:

- First remove anything that is choking your life force: this might be over-activity, difficult interpersonal situations, self-stressing attitudes, and so on.
- In the second phase, look to see where in the garden the new life is emerging, and encourage this growth. This is the phase of therapy when you spend time focusing on what is right about you, reminding yourself of what gives you pleasure and really makes your heart sing, and receiving the encouragement and support you need to blossom in your true colours.
- In the third phase, we must look again at the garden to see whether there are any earthworks that need to be done – putting in a new feature, or moving existing plants to more appropriate places. In therapy, this is the time when you may want to look at some of the deeper issues that have been thwarting your potential and progress in life. It may also be the time when you want to contemplate making bigger life changes, such as changing your job or moving house, or perhaps sorting out a difficult, dysfunctional relationship.

The point of reminding you of this staged approach is that it is important to be wise about the timing and pace of any changes you make: you need to take into account the state of your physical health and the strength of the foundations you have laid inside yourself through your earlier therapy to ensure that a particular change is a good one.

It is important to ensure that change is being made for the right reasons, and that you are not merely running away from some aspect of yourself. In Alcoholics Anonymous meetings they call this 'doing a geographical', which means thinking that a problem can be solved by moving away from it physically rather than by tackling it on the psychological level. While physical moves may be required in the long term (as can be seen in stage three of our garden analogy), it is usually better to start with the work of sorting out the ways you are stressing or distressing yourself first – by working through stages one and two – otherwise you are likely to take these problems with you wherever you go.

A time will come when you realize you have reached a new level of stability and health, and at this stage it begins to feel possible to embark upon the regular practice of self-help. At this point the need for your therapy sessions begins to diminish. Your therapists will help to guide you in deciding when it is an appropriate time to stop therapy. Energy therapists in acupuncture and shiatsu will be able to tell you when the body's energies are back into better balance; soon you will learn to know how this feels, and so be able to recognize when it is necessary to go back for 'top-up' sessions. It is certainly hoped that, by this time, your life and health will be on a very much sounder footing, and that you will be experiencing the strong benefits of all the learning changes and self-discovery that you have made.

If you have been to the Bristol Cancer Help Centre, attending the two follow-up days will give you an invaluable boost to your motivation and morale. You will meet others who are further down the path than you, and they will by now be showing the benefits of sticking to their programme. You will also be surprised at how far your personal goalposts have moved, and how much you are now able to fine-tune your programme and goals.

Regardless of whether or not you are able to come to the Centre and take part directly in the therapy programme, it is important to give yourself recognition for what you have achieved through adopting the Bristol Approach, and to have your progress recognized by the therapists who see you regularly. Embarking upon the holistic way of doing things is not the easy option; it would be far easier to stick your head in the sand or get on with 'life as normal'. It is therefore very good to take stock regularly so that you can really honour yourself for the work you have done and the progress you are making.

7
Making Self-help Work for You: Psychoneuroimmunology in Practice

This chapter returns to the crucial linkages between mind, body and spirit in achieving and maintaining health and well-being. It explores in detail the therapeutic practice of relaxation, meditation, visualization and affirmation – all of which you can learn to do on your own, and all of which can produce the beneficial effects in the neurological system that are so powerful in restoring and preserving physical health.

When You're Ready . . .

This chapter contains exercises and plenty of practical information to assist you in developing your own programme of self-nurturing therapy to enhance your healing response. You may find it helpful at this stage to return to Chapter 2, 'Science and the Bristol Approach', to remind yourself of the very real benefits to your internal physiology that these techniques can bring about. Not only are they enjoyable once you grasp them, they are enormously good for you, too.

Before going any further, it is worth repeating that it will be almost impossible to embark successfully on any form of self-help if your energy levels are very low – by which we mean below the 30 per cent line marked in Figure 6 (p. 42) as part of the energy model. So it is important to be realistic about whether you are yet in a position to start and sustain self-help activity. If you have a good supporter who can do lots of the work for you, or a therapist who can support you as you learn some of the techniques, it may be that you can begin to try out some of the approaches described here even before you restore your energy levels; alternatively, it may be better for you to concentrate first on resting and addressing the energy deficit. Even so, you may wish to start reading about and familiarizing yourself with these techniques; to do so may give you further encouragement to get to the points where you can apply them fully and reap the benefits.

When you decide you have the strength and the stamina to get going, it is likely that you'll find it hugely satisfying to not always be so reliant on others to lead you to a place of peace and tranquillity.

Endorphins: The Healing Messengers

Central to psychoneuroimmunology (PNI) is the principle, now endorsed by scientific studies, that changes in mental and emotional state can bring about changes in physical well-being. At the heart of the process are the endorphins – chemical messengers that are released by the body as a result of a pleasurable event. These create a state of relaxation in which we feel safe, happy and filled with goodwill – a state that promotes health and balance in the body. Crucially, this response occurs whether we actually have the experience or just imagine it, the body being unable to distinguish between reality and its mental/emotional image; so it makes very good sense to enable ourselves to bring about the response through our imaginative powers.

The following exercise, developed by our senior doctor Sara Miller, is a good introduction to the way in which you can activate the PNI response yourself.

- Think of an animal which makes you laugh. Think of it as many times a day as possible, finding a picture or other *aide-mémoire* which you can put in a prominent place to remind you (maybe the fridge door).
- Make lists of people, places, pets, activities, which you find especially pleasurable, which bring a smile to your face when you recall them. Choose one or two from each list every day to remember as often as possible, especially if you are feeling low. Go to sleep thinking of them, and bring them to mind as you wake.
- Recall happy events and times in your life. Write them down and relive them, letting a smile come to your lips.
- If you are in pain, imagine one of your favourite 'positive triggers' (e.g. a pet), encouraging endorphin production and reducing the pain.

Creating Sacred Space for Self-healing

When you begin to apply self-healing approaches, such as meditation, relaxation, visualization and affirmation, it is often very beneficial to have a place or spot to go to that is dedicated entirely to this self-healing work, and for your own personal prayer and quiet reflection. In this way routine and familiarity help us to create time and space for ourselves that foster a force or environment for healing to take place. You are more likely to make a commitment to your daily practice if you don't have to run around finding somewhere quiet to do it.

Space in our homes and gardens may be plentiful or limited. However, if you can find even a small place that is your own, it is a wonderful chance to set up a space that takes on the intention of healing; it will renew you and help you in your daily practices and help you to set up a healing routine.

So, find a place where you can keep a chair or meditation stool. Add a small table on which you can place meaningful things – maybe a candle, a plant or flowers, along with a favourite picture, a book of inspiration and possibly some pieces from nature such as shells, stones or crystals, a shawl or blanket to keep you warm, and any other objects that you associate with health, happiness, joy, healing and images of the future.

This is your place, one that will encourage and support you.

Relaxation

'Everything you do can be done better from a place of relaxation.'[62]

Learning relaxation can initially be likened to reducing the idling speed on an engine that is revving too fast and therefore wasting precious fuel. If you are full of tension then a great deal of your precious vital energy is being wasted. This is especially true during the frightening period of diagnosis and the lead-up to treatment, as well as during and after treatment.

If relaxation exercises and techniques are new to you they can seem quite difficult and maybe even daunting at first. Most of us live very busy lives, and finding time to fit in relaxation so that it can be of most benefit needs careful thought and planning. Also, when we are feeling unwell, or afraid, or out of control of so much of our life, the thought of slowing down and letting go may be quite difficult. Nevertheless, patience, support from experienced others, and finding the right relaxation method or approach for your unique and individual lifestyle and personality will prove effective in the long run.

It is important to understand that there are many approaches to relaxation and many ways of achieving it; it will be helpful to take advice on the differences and then to experiment for yourself. In the first instance you will probably gain more by using an approach that is led and guided by an experienced, professionally trained person. This way you can start by being relaxed passively by someone else – a relaxation therapist, yoga teache, or hypnotherapist – talking you through or teaching you a relaxation exercise. You can then follow this up at home by listening to the tape or CD of the exercise or approach they took with you.

Relaxation can also be achieved by movement of the body, for instance in learning yoga, which combines gentle movement with deep relaxation and meditation practices. You can also receive touch to soften and release the tension in the body through massage, with or without aromatherapy; healing by laying on of hands; and shiatsu. These therapies will enable you to experience what relaxation feels like so that you know what you are aiming for.

You can use two or more approaches for fuller experiences. Our body needs change, and it is good to have a range of approaches at our disposal in order to respond to our changing nature and needs.

To find a relaxation therapist in your area you can contact the organization Relaxation for Living, which trains relaxation therapists; the contact number is given in Appendix 2. Many treatment centres and local health centres include complementary therapies and relaxation classes. Specialist information about local support groups, including relaxation classes, and other complementary therapists is available from hospitals, clinics, treatment centres and nurses. Self-help support groups often have very experienced leaders or facilitators, and they too can guide you to find a suitably qualified person to help you find the best way for you to experience relaxation.

In addition, many local education programmes offer day-time and evening relaxation classes. You can also find leaflets on local classes and practitioners in libraries and healthfood shops. It may be helpful to contact the organization Relaxation for Living to see if there is a group in your area. The Yoga for Health Foundation offers residential courses, for beginners upwards, including week-long residential courses in yoga for people with or recovering from cancer. (For contact details see Appendix 2.)

If the relaxation therapist does not provide you with notes or a prepared tape or CD, ask their permission to tape-record the session, for use at home. You can also ask them to recommend books, other tapes and videos or DVDs. Your supporter may wish to come along to your relaxation session to learn how to talk you into a relaxed state. What some people have done to great effect, having learnt the principles, is to make a tape of their own voice talking through a relaxation exercise. It is wonderful to hear your own voice telling you to relax and let go. This forms a great template for your new healing relationship with yourself.

Relaxation takes time to perfect. The benefits tend to be cumulative, and initially you may not relax profoundly. However, with daily practice the process soon becomes part of your natural self and begins to have a deepening, positive and restorative effect.

Do not be surprised if you fall asleep when you first start to practise relaxation. Usually, when we first start the process, we quickly become aware of how absolutely exhausted we are beneath our 'coping façade'. Eventually, as your energy levels are raised, this will stop happening and you will be able to stay awake throughout the relaxation.

It is worth emphasizing at this point that sleep is not the same as relaxation. Many people believe that falling asleep in a chair is the same as relaxing. The reality is that despite the sleep, we can wake up as anxious as before: this is evident from analysis that has shown that levels of the substances produced by the stress chemicals in our urine can be as high after sleep as they were before. So even if you are able to sleep, it is also very important to learn relaxation.

Exercise: Relaxation

Here is a simple exercise to help you to fully relax your body.

- Close your eyes, remove glasses, loosen tight clothing and take your shoes off.
- Start by adjusting your position so that you are sitting comfortably. Don't cross your legs, ankles or feet, or hands; just sit with your back supported. If your legs are too short to reach the floor comfortably, then put a book or bag on the floor on which to rest your feet. Lie on the floor if you wish.
- There may be sounds in the room, or outside; remember that life goes on and that we can become relaxed despite the noises around us. Just let the noises be there, and do not be distracted if they come.
- Raise your shoulders up to your ears and let them fall down gently.
- Open your mouth as if yawning, close it a little and rock your lower jaw left and right.
- Close your mouth and push your tongue hard up to the roof of your mouth. Let the tongue spring back. Loosen your jaw some more.
- Once again raise your shoulders to your ears, then release them gently.
- Now just breathe normally and softly.
- Allow your inward breath to become a little deeper.
- As you breathe, just notice the breath and bring your attention to the sensation of the breath flowing at the tip

of your nostrils.

- Now notice the natural gentle movement of your chest as you breathe in and breathe out.
- Take a deep breath without straining.
- Allow the breath to come and go effortlessly.
- Just continue for a moment or two longer.
- Keep the gentle awareness of the natural rise and fall of your breath to help you to soften and relax and remove any tiredness or tension.
- Take your attention to your feet.
- As you breathe in, imagine or allow your inward breath to soften the texture and feel of your feet . . .
- . . . while your outward breath takes away any tiredness or tension.
- Do the same with your lower legs.
- Inward breath brings softness and relaxation . . .
- . . . outward breath removes tiredness.
- Now your upper legs . . .
- Inward softening – relaxing . . .
- . . . outward – taking away tension.
- Now your lower back . . .
- Now your shoulders . . .
- Now your arms and hands . . .
- Now into your chest and abdomen . . .
- Up into your neck, head, scalp and face . . .
- Continue to breathe slowly and peacefully.
- Check around your body. Is there any remaining tension or tiredness? If so, take your breath there to soften and renew.

Allow yourself to rest in this position for as long as you can. You may even fall asleep. When you are ready to return to your day, gently move to an upright sitting position.

It is important not to rush; take your time over whatever you might have to do now. The relaxation response continues to work if you don't rush about after the exercise.

Meditation

When you first begin meditation you will learn that to have a simple but effective relaxation exercise will help you to achieve a more effective meditation practice. So learn how to slow the body, thought processes and senses down, in order to let go and move into the quieter places found deeply within you. Also, if you are a beginner at both relaxation and meditation, consider the benefits of joining a group, for support, learning and fun.

As with relaxation, when starting meditation we have to accept that the world isn't silent and that there is no real external haven, free from distraction. Stress and strain will still be potentially in our lives, but the process and accumulative effect of meditation, again as with relaxation, helps us to reduce our level of arousal and allows us to stay connected to the stiller parts of our being and connected to the natural healing process within us. By taking a few minutes every day to meditate we can gradually change our perception of our lives and learn to respond in healthier and positive ways.

There are many approaches to meditation. Some are located within religious practice, for example in Christianity, Judaism, Buddhism and other religious traditions. Equally, there are other ways and means of learning meditation that do not have a religious focus.

When seeking a meditation class, course, group or teacher it is important for you to establish on what basis the meditation practice is set. You can find out about local meditation groups through the same sources as for relaxation. In some instances fees are minimal, in other cases meditation courses and programmes are more detailed and dedicated to a specific set of meditation practices and may require higher fees. You will need to pose your questions around what you can expect and what is expected of you before embarking on a commitment to your chosen approach.

Meditation does not have to be expensive in terms of fees or time. What is important is to feel comfortable with what you are doing and how you are doing it, and to make the commitment to yourself to engage in this potentially profound self-healing approach.

Exercise: Healing Meditation

- Find a comfortable place to sit, with your back straight and your feet firmly on the ground. Try to ensure that you will not be disturbed during your meditation by taking the phone off the hook or putting the answering machine on.
- Take about five minutes to relax your body completely, working through from the feet up to the head. Imagine that you can just let go of all the muscles; feel them soften and release, allowing the tension to flow out of your whole being.
- Focus particularly on the stomach, the shoulders and the jaw, as these are areas where we often, without realizing it, hold a great deal of tension in the muscles.
- When your body feels totally relaxed, bring your attention to your breathing. Don't try to change it; just be aware of the breath moving in and out of your body.
- Notice as much as you can about your breathing, such as how it feels as the breath moves in and out of the nostrils and where you take the breath to in your body. Stay with this for another five minutes or so.
- Now imagine that you are outside in the sunshine, try to get a sense of the light of the sun, warm but not too hot, and shining down on you. You might like to imagine that you are lying on a quiet beach soaking up the sunlight. Imagine that you can breathe in the light of the sun, taking it into your body. Let the light fill up every cell of your body, as if you are drinking in light. When you feel glowing and full of light, let that light move anywhere in your body where you feel that you are in need of healing. Feel your cells transforming, becoming energized as the

Basic self-healing: lifting your spirits
This is a meditation to lift your spirits, developed by the senior healer at the Bristol Cancer Help Centre, Janet Swan.

For each of us there is a place that we remember because it had that special quality, the ability to lift our spirits. This may be a church or a temple, a forest or hilltop, a bluebell wood or seashore. We remember it, as a place we felt expanded and joyful.

Here is a way to go there, at any time you want.

- Find a quiet place and close your eyes.
- Relax the body and take three gentle breaths.
- Now find your own quiet centre within.
- Remind yourself of your special place where you felt quietened, expanded and in awe.
- Take yourself fully there – feel the atmosphere and use your senses to really *be* there, sensing smells, colours and sounds.
- Lift your mind to contact your higher self. Call upon spiritual helpers, whether God, angels, the Spirit of Life, the spirit of the place or nature.
- Stay quiet, allowing yourself to fully feel and expand that context into a higher state of consciousness until the spiritual energy has filled and recharged you.
- When ready, release and return, taking time to integrate all you have experienced.

radiance heals and restores you.
- Now let the light expand out as if you are radiating light into the energy fields around your body, so that you are imagining yourself glowing with light and health. Stay with this part of the meditation for about ten minutes, really using your imagination to help you.
- Now bring your attention back to the breath, silently saying, every time you breathe in, 'I am breathing health,' and on each out-breath saying to yourself, 'I am completely relaxed.' As you do this, feel the truth of what

you are saying, and believe it so that it becomes a reality for you.

- Now let it all go and bring yourself back to the room, slowly and gently. Feel the ground beneath your feet and become aware once more of your surroundings.

Visualization

'Dream your dream, focus your intention, and take each step to make it real.'[63]

'The use of imagery is considered to help us to form a bridge between our inner and outer worlds, our conscious minds and our unconscious minds.'[64]

Visualization is the creation of thoughts, images and pictures within the mind and through the imagination. The visualization can include the following of a storyline, which may be quite vivid and clear; or it may be more of a sense of movement or colour, and may include your senses of hearing, smell and even touch. The storyline may be one that is completely made up, or the recall of something that has happened to you to or others. Visualization can be very personal and private, developed on your own; or it can be guided by someone who is assisting you, either in person or by your listening to a recording. In the latter case, the process can be one-to-one, or in some instances it may be within a small group of people sharing similar issues or current life situations. Visualization does not have to rely exclusively on successfully drawing a picture in the imagination; often it may be more of a memory, or just holding on to the intention to recall or revisit a situation in order to bring about the desired response. Visualization is a potentially powerful self-help and self-healing process.

You can develop a personalized visualization on your own,

for yourself, but it is often more successful, certainly for the beginner, to work on it with the support and guidance of another, ideally a professional who is trained and experienced in the use of imagery work (which can include visualization, guided imagery, and how to develop personal affirmations). Such a person can help you make sure that your chosen visualization/ image/affirmation is as complete and as appropriate as possible.

Professional practitioners of visualization techniques are often trained in counselling skills. Indeed, they may be working as counsellors or psychotherapists and, as part of their practice, using the often untapped depths of the imagination and deeper mind or unconscious. However, it is also possible for those who have been trained in relaxation techniques, or hypnosis, to be competent and helpful in this insightful process.

To find a suitable practitioner, you can look in all the places noted above in the section on relaxation. If there does not seem to be anyone available who is trained in this work, then there are books and audio-visual materials that can give you practical help to start with. A suggested list of books can be found in Appendix 3, 'Further Reading'.

Much of the pre-recorded material leads you through a visualization which is term-guided. This means that the voice of the guide leads you on a general journey, rather than a specific journey to suit your own personal needs. You listen to (and/or watch) the tape, and the voice of the guide leads you through a very pleasant imagery journey. The aim of this type of visualization can be to demonstrate how to build up a picture, or to help you to relax: both are important and can enable you to build confidence and feel the benefits of imagery work.

Through visualization we create a scenario that requires us to be alive, well and present in the future. We effectively undo negative feelings and fears that may have arisen within us as a result of being given a life-threatening diagnosis of cancer – relating, for example, to the powerful messages you might have received about how long you are likely to survive.

Through personal visualization or imagery, you can help yourself not only to stimulate a healing response to your cancer, but also to gain messages from the body about what is going on within it: it becomes a two-way process during which you form a deeper relationship with the body and stop to listen and feel what the body needs to say. Developing your capacity to use imagery in this way will help the body to cope better – especially during all forms of cancer treatment, and afterwards when you are recovering from treatment, but also into the future, in maintaining your health and overall well-being.

When you are preparing yourself to find an image or visualization plan to help in the removal of your cancer and the rebuilding of a healthy body there are a number of things to consider.

1 Preparation is everything. Take time to think about the image. It is important that you feel comfortable with the image and have not taken on one that does not suit your personality or beliefs. For instance, you may not feel happy with one that is aggressive, such as sharks racing through your system attacking and killing cancer cells. If so, you might select an image that is more peaceful while still being efficient, e.g. a fairy or dwarf who picks up the cells and carries them to the kidneys to be washed away; or light that transforms the cells so that they dissolve or disappear.

2 Write your image down, or draw it, until you feel that this is one that you would like to use.

3 Ask others for their suggestions too.

4 Before you start to use your image in relation to removing the cancer, have a few 'practice runs'. Take the time to relax and bring your image to your mind's eye; see the image in as much detail as possible, then expand it so that it can go throughout your body. When you feel that you can comfortably call your image to mind at will, then you

can start to use it in the removal or control of your cancer.

5 It is important to note that images can change. You might carry on using the same one you start with; but with practice and time you might feel you wish to refine or change it. Stay open-minded; if it does not seem to be working, then you might have selected an image that you are not totally comfortable with, or one that is too complicated.

6 Images are very personal, too; some people will be capable of creating very detailed and exact images, while others use less defined images. Both ways are valid and capable of working successfully.

Visualization for Healing Cells in the Body

- Imagine that you are approaching a beautiful waterfall that is cascading gently into a shallow, placid lake. You come closer to this deep, healing blue . . . the perfect iridescent blue of the rainbow, full of light and colour.

- You wade into the soft, warm pool of water until you are directly beneath the flow of this gentle waterfall. Feel how soft and cool and healing this beautiful blue water is as it pours over your body, soothing and nourishing every part of you, washing away all your tiredness, all your fears.

- Feel each and every drop as it begins to penetrate through the top of your head. Guide it down, down, down, until it reaches your heart, healing and comforting it. Feel this cool, healing blue water as it enters your bloodstream, pumped through each cell in your body, cleansing, calming, cooling and balancing every cell, every nerve, every fibre of your body.

- Feel it as it is flowing through you now . . . through your shoulders, down your arms to your fingertips, back up to your elbows, back to your chest, into your lungs, into your heart.

- This cool, blue, healing light and water is now flowing

down through your stomach, cooling and restoring all of
the organs in your abdomen, your digestive system, down
through your hips, your thighs, your knees, your calves,
your ankles and your toes.

- Now you see this blue light penetrating each and every cell
of your body. Feel it as it is cleansing and refreshing every
cell . . . healing every cell . . . making each one well,
healthy and whole . . . well, healthy and whole. Complete.
- You are now one with the placid lake. You are as placid,
calm and peaceful as the lake. Allow the healing to flow
through you. Allow yourself to be a calm, cool, blue drop
in the placid lake.
- You are one with the lake, you are well, healthy, whole
and complete. You are one with the lake, flowing down,
cleansing every cell . . . see every cell as new, healthy, well
and whole.

Each and every time that you listen to these words it will reinforce the healing.

You might like to tape-record your own voice so that you
can passively listen, just following the guidelines until you are
confident with the sequences. You may find that, with experience, you go on to refine the details on the tape; or you might
find that you do not need it any longer. However, on some days
you might not have the same level of energy as on others, and
the tape can be a good standby if you need to return to listening and following at these times.

Grounding Visualization

This visualization can be used at the beginning of your day. It
can also be useful when you are preparing for hospital treatments. It helps to balance our awareness by bringing together
our thoughts, feelings and sensations, particularly when we are
feeling 'scattered' or anxious or in pain.

Again, you might like to tape-record your own voice so

that you can listen and follow the guidelines until you are more confident.

Remember to be gentle, and do not overexert yourself. Your breaths need to follow what you are capable of doing; over-emphasizing the breath can make you dizzy. So pace yourself to your own comfort level.

Everyone will have their own personal experience of this visualization. For some people it will be relatively easy to imagine or create an image; others may not see a picture or image at all, but respond more by physically sensing the area on which the focus is developed. So when the words 'visualize' or 'imagine' or 'feel' or 'send' are used, find the one that relates to you; there is no right or wrong way.

- Sit comfortably.
- Gently check your body and make adjustments as needed to your posture, so that you are not distracted by discomfort caued by poor positioning or lack of support for your body.
- Take your awareness to your breath. Notice where you move your chest as you breathe in – does the front of your chest move, your back, or sides?
- Breathe in, pause just for a moment then breathe out. Before you breathe in again, just pause for another moment; then breathe. Do this for three or four breaths.
- Relax and breathe naturally without pausing between breaths.
- Now sink into your seat more – slowing down and letting go more and more.
- Take a gentle deep breath in; raise your shoulders; breathe out and drop your shoulders. Do this three more times.
- Loosen your jaw – rocking the jaw left to right a few times will help.
- Allow yourself to soften more, slowing down and letting go more and more.

- Take your awareness to your lower abdomen, below your navel.
- The life force of energy is in this place.
- Allow yourself to connect with this space.
- As you make the connection you might be able to see it, or create an image, or just physically sense it. Bring your awareness to this source of personal energy.
- Begin to release some of the vital personal energy: send some of the energy down through your pelvis, directing it down each leg.
- Continue to flow the energy down your legs and out through the soles of your feet.
- Continue to send the energy, down and down, deeply into the earth, passing underground rocks, rivers and plant life.
- Feel the energy deeply penetrating the earth.
- Find a place within the earth to bring your energy to.
- Now allow the energy to spread out and form fibres or threads which anchor themselves to the earth, firmly rooted.
- Now allow the anchored or rooted fibres to stay fixed, but to become hollow tubes.
- Through the rooted tubes, now draw on the healing and grounding life force of the earth's energy.
- Begin to draw up through the tubes the earth's energies.
- Bring the energy up and into your lower abdomen, the place that you started from.
- Mix the earth's energy with your own – blending, strengthening your energy.
- Allow the energy to rise up to your heart and to be pumped around your body.
- Send the energy up and out through the top of your head and allow it to fall down and around you – like a shower or fountain.
- This shower finds its way back into the earth. You are now held in this blended energy field.

- The energy, as it falls gently over you and into the earth, is then united underneath your feet. Close and seal the energy under your feet and feel safe and nurtured by this blended energy, the earth's and your own, which is serving to ground, nourish and protect you, balancing and holding you safely together.
- Relax and return to wakefulness when you are ready.

'The Cloak of Light'
This is another self-healing visualization technique from our senior healer, Janet Swan.

- Find a quiet place, and close your eyes.
- Relax the body, and take three gentle breaths.
- Now find your own quiet centre within.
- Focus your awareness on your heart.
- Imagine a golden, healing light falling around you.
- Allow this light to fill and surround your body like a cloak of light.
- Hold this image for as long as you need.
- When ready, draw this cloak closely around you, breathe more deeply and open your eyes.

This simple exercise enables you to remember yourself and reconnect to the universal life force whenever you need to. It takes the mind away from outer pressures, and gives it a healing task to do. Drawing the cloak of light closely around you at the finish means that you contain the good effects and have extra protection afterwards. With practice, this exercise can be done almost anywhere, at any time you need.

How to Create a Personal Image
If personal imagery work appeals to you, it will be important to find an image of the cancer itself. This might include visualizing what the cancer looks like to you – its nature, its colour or tex-

ture – and where in the body you see or imagine it to be. This, of course, does not have to be biologically accurate. Some people have seen their cancers as blocks of ice or spiky conkers, others as specks of sand or lumps of jelly. It is entirely up to you.

Having done this, you will need to find an image of the agent or helper that you believe is capable of shrinking the cancer in your body. It is important to make sure that the agent or helper you choose is something you feel comfortable with and something that you can believe in as actually strong enough to assist in the healing process. In the next section of the chapter you will find examples of visualizations and images that others have found helpful.

After you have found the image for your cancer and that of the helper/agent, it is important that you also seek to create a positive picture or feeling of yourself as whole and healed. This can sometimes be helped along by also seeing yourself in the future at some event that you are looking forward to or really want to attend. In other words, you include in the visualization the presence of yourself alive and well in the future.

Every time you use this visualization, make sure that in your mind's eye the cancer is all gone.

Bringing Imagery into Your Daily Life and Treatment

The following suggestions offer ways in which you can use imagery to help you with your situation and improve your quality of life. This is not an exhaustive list. As mentioned above, it is important to find an image that you feel comfortable with; you might find that the image changes with time and experience. As you become competent with the image, gaining in ability to create images that are helpful to your own situation and needs, your confidence will also increase.

Remember that images can be made up of memories, or images that come to you through your other senses; these might include feelings, memories in your body and its sensation, thoughts without pictures, and sounds.

Talk your ideas through with others, and be willing to borrow others' ideas until you can find your own images. Don't worry about getting it all absolutely perfect at first; just make a regular commitment and practise. At first you might find that you can do the imagery work only for a short time – most people start off with five to ten minutes once or twice a day, and build it up from there.

Remember that preparation is 50 per cent of success. If you are using imagery work at the time of having surgery, chemotherapy or radiotherapy, then do your best to practise your imagery work before the treatment starts. If possible, explain in advance to the health professionals who are treating you that you are using this self-help approach, and ask for their help in ensuring that you can use the technique during your treatment. You might need to explain how they can best support you – for example, allowing you a few minutes to settle yourself or to turn on a tape-recorder of the imagery if that is what you need. This will give them time to help you to do this and to arrange practical matters such as making available an electric socket or extension lead.

If you are nervous, you might make yourself a tape of your own voice; again, seek health professionals' support and practical help in setting up your tape-player ahead of the treatment starting. It will only take a few minutes to have it there.

When at home, too, remember to let others know not to disturb you while you are doing your imagery/visualizations.

Now here are some suggestions of images that others have found helpful.

Images of breath   As you breathe in deeply, the healing breath energy is taken deep into the lungs, where it enters the bloodstream and is taken all around the body. The healthy cells are strengthened and nourished. As you breathe out, the diseased cells dissolve and leave the body.

Images of helpers/agents The following are suggestions of images that some have found helpful.

- *Sharks*: as they go along they find the cancer cells and eat them or tear them up.
- *Fantasy* or *fairytale small creatures*, such as fairies or elves, or cartoon characters like the Seven Dwarfs, who collect the cancer cells and either take them carefully to the kidneys to be flushed away, or place them in some solution which makes them dissolve or renders them harmless.
- *Soldiers* or *warriors* who, on finding the cells, render them helpless or destroy them altogether.
- A *particular warrior* or *knight* who rides through the body, on a horse, carrying a lance, spearing away the cells.
- *Heroes* within a vessel, e.g. a tiny submarine, that sails around the body removing the cancer cells.
- *Significant characters from stories* who you consider have strength of purpose and bring change by their strength and determination, helping your body to remove all of those cells that do not allow you to be healthy and whole. You can create a storyline.
- *Significant religious people* or events which have meaning for you.
- *Angels* and other helpful beings.

Images of light and colour Immense power can be represented by light and colour that are individually meaningful and wonderful to see. This light and colour can often be imagined, or experienced, as richer, stronger and more expansive than those we are used to seeing in our everyday life.

The light and colour are seen to flood the body, removing impurities and dissolving the cancer cells.

Light and colour images include:

- *Sun*: sunlight has been used extensively in the past to help

cure TB and skin diseases.
- *Golden light*: imagine a beam of golden light pouring down, entering the crown of the head and flowing through the body in a healing golden stream. Imagine that the diseased cells cannot survive the intensity of the light; they begin to shrivel and die off.
- *Pure white light.*
- *Rainbow light and coloured light.*
- *Favourite colours.*
- *Waterfalls of colour and light.*
- *Laser beams.*

Personal images   Images can also be developed from those things that are familiar and hold personal importance; for example, they are often taken from everyday life and hobbies. A couple of examples are:

- A *magic hoover*, travelling round the body sucking up cancer cells.
- *Bulldog clips* that clamp themselves on all the blood vessels that the tumour has created to feed itself, thereby cutting off its food supply.

Images from nature   Popular and effective natural images include:

- *Water* that is perceived as cleansing – waterfalls, lakes, sea, showers.
- *Flowers* that put down whole and healthy seeds which unearth the cancer cells and cause them to die.
- *Animals* – either real or fantasy – coming to sniff out and destroy cancer cells.
- *Snowflakes*, falling and freezing the cancer cells out.
- *Ice*: the cancer may be seen as a block of ice that gradually melts.

- *Strong trees*, sending shoots or roots to strengthen the body and to remove the cancer cells that are in the way of the tree.
- *The wind*, coming to clean throughout the body, moving as a warm and brisk breeze throughout the whole body, taking away the cancer cells, which are likened to dead wood or dried-up leaves, and whisking them away.
- *Piranha/catfish* that can be released into the body every so often to swim around and eat up any cells that are sick or damaged.

Images of the treatment itself These may be particularly useful during or following radiotherapy or chemotherapy.

- See the rays of radiotherapy as destroying the cancer cells only, while protecting the healthy cells.
- See chemotherapy surging around the body, but again affecting only the cancer cells.

Images of music Hearing, seeing or feeling the music that is important and pleasurable for you can be immensely powerful. As the notes flow within you, they fill all the body with pleasure, creating harmony, setting up new cells, and removing the cancer cells. Different notes may be chosen that melt away the cancer cells, with other notes renewing and making new healthy cells. The cancer is simply dissolved away. (See the box on p. 199 for some suggestions of music that may help you in your self-healing work.)

Affirmations

Talking to ourselves is very important. Just as we see and visualize things through the mind's eye, so it is not unusual for us to talk to ourselves through our mind's voice to help us in our motivations and to provide comfort and reassurance in times of stress or

Basic self-healing: hands on

Why not try this exercise, developed by our senior healer Janet Swan, designed to help you awake your own healing abilities?

To a certain extent we are *all* healers. While healers are trained to develop, focus and direct the healing energy more strongly, we all have the ability to call upon this power to come to us from the universal life force for our own benefit. Try awakening this energy with your own hands.

- Find a quiet place and close your eyes.
- Relax the body and take three gentle breaths.
- Then rub your hands together briskly for about 15 seconds.
- Now call upon the healing light from the source to come through your heart to your hands.
- Place your hands on any part of your body in need and allow the healing to flow through.
- When you sense completion, place your hands back on your lap and sit quietly, breathing gently, until you are ready to move.

strain. Within the world of healing and self-awareness this form of self-encouragement is often termed 'affirmation'. To *affirm* something is to make a positive, durable and believable statement to fit in with what we wish for or want to create; a statement which reflects what we value and uphold as good, and supports our healing process. Affirmations can be used to supplement and complement imagery and healing visualizations. For those people who find that they do not want to visualize, or to whom imagery work does not appeal, affirmations offer an alternative route.

The key to the success of an affirming, self-healing sentence or phrase is the ability to build an affirmation that is carefully constructed in your own words, of a manageable length – something which is not overly long and wordy and at the same time upholds your beliefs and values for yourself.

How to Apply and Use Your Personal Affirmation

- Compose and write down your affirmation.
- Sit comfortably and say your affirmation out loud. Notice how you feel when you say the words. Do they feel appropriate, or at least acceptable and believable for the time being? It is not unusual to change the affirmation with use, when you have gained confidence or have a better sense of what you are trying to achieve or want for yourself.
- Affirmations can be written out and put in obvious places to remind you to say or think about them when you see them. Stick the affirmation on your mirror, on the back of your diary, on your computer screen or bedside table; have it on display in the place you go to relax and meditate.
- People vary as to when they say or think about their affirmations. Some say them when they first get up in the morning and repeat them at particular times again during the day. Other people fit their affirmation into the time when they are relaxing, saying the affirmation when they have reached a relaxed state in which they are open and receptive to the words and sentiments. Affirmations can also be slotted in before or after meditation.
- The affirmation is usually said a few times at each chosen moment; this helps to endorse it and to establish in yourself an attachment to it and what you are aiming for.

Suggestions for Affirmations

Prior to and during conventional cancer treatments

'I see myself responding positively to the healing effects of radiotherapy/surgery/chemotherapy.'

'My body and whole self are responding well to the treatments.'

'Only the cancer is being affected by the treatment, the rest of my body is safe and healthy.'

'I believe that this treatment is healing me.'

Music to aid self-healing: classical moods

Quiet, meditative
Copland: *Quiet City* (10 minutes)
Chopin: Nocturnes for solo piano (4–6 minutes each)
Bach: Concerto for two violins, 2nd movement (7 minutes)
Beethoven: Piano Concerto No. 3, 2nd movement (8 minutes)
Bizet: *Carmen*, Act III Entr'acte (3 minutes)

Images
Frank Bridge: *The Sea* (20 minutes)
Debussy: Preludes for solo piano (5 minutes each)
Debussy: Three Nocturnes (5–10 minutes each)
Elgar: *The Wand of Youth*, suites 1 and 2 (several
    movements, 3–5 minutes each)
Elgar: *Dream Children* (6 minutes)

Uplifting, inspirational
Brahms: Violin Concerto (40 minutes)
Borodin: Overture, *Prince Igor* (10 minutes)
Bizet: Symphony in C (20 minutes)
Bizet: *L'Arlesienne*, suites 1 and 2 (several movements, 4–7
    minutes each)
Grieg: *Holberg Suite* (20 minutes)

Musical journeys
Borodin: In the Steppes of Central Asia (8 minutes)
Copland: Appalachian Springs (25 minutes)
Sibelius: En Saga (15 minutes)
Mendelssohn: Symphony No. 4, 'Italian' (20 minutes)
Beethoven: Piano Sonata No. 26 in E flat

Pastoral
Butterworth: *The Banks of Green Willow* (7 minutes)
Butterworth: *Two English Idylls* (6 minutes each)
Vaughan Williams: *The Lark Ascending* (15 minutes)
Beethoven: Symphony No. 6, 'Pastoral' (45 minutes)
Finzi: Romance for string orchestra (10 minutes)

General affirmations
'I see myself well, whole and healthy.'
'My body is responding to my healing interventions.'
'Every day I see myself well and happy and free of cancer.'
'I am strong and healthy and see my body as well and balanced.'

For the future
'I know that I have a positive future ahead of me.'
'I am strong today and will be gaining strength and health as each day passes.'
'I see myself well and happy and enjoying my daughter's graduation next summer.'
'I can feel the excitement and health building in my body as I prepare for my holidays next year.'
'I see myself holding my new grandchildren in the future.'

8
Supporting the Supporters

This chapter looks at the particular challenges facing those who are close to, and care for, people with cancer. It suggests what their particular needs might be, and how these can be met with greatest benefit both to themselves and those for whom they are caring, in a point-by-point 'Supporter Survival Plan'.

At the Bristol Cancer Help Centre we have had the opportunity of asking people with serious illness which of their traumatic life events they feel have most affected their own health. A very frequent reply has been looking after a relative or close person with cancer or other serious illness. This alerted us to the vulnerability of those who are in the supporting role, and led in 1998 to a change of policy: to offer places on the Centre's courses for people in the supporting role on an exactly equal footing to those they are caring for.

In the past, supporters of people with cancer were always invited to attend the Bristol Cancer Help Centre with their friend or partner with cancer, but this was in a passive role. The main reason for the supporters' being there was to help to provide any practical help that was needed, and to gather new information and learn the various self-help skills in order to reinforce the practice of the person with cancer once they got home. The Centre did also run groups within all of its courses for supporters to begin to explore their state and needs; however, it became clear that this was really just scratching the surface of the problem – that in reality the supporters needed counselling, healing, bodywork and even appointments with doctors in their own right.

(At Bristol, we see supporters who stand in many relationships to the person whom they are supporting: close family members, spouses, lovers, colleagues, friends. For simplicity's sake, in this chapter we use the word 'partner' to denote both individuals in the supporting relationship, irrespective of the nature of their personal relationship.)

Complex Feelings

Many supporters suffer from acute anxiety or intense grief, not to mention confusion about the complex set of feelings they are experiencing. While wishing dearly to 'get it right' for loved ones, many are troubled by feelings of guilt because, underneath a reasonably calm exterior, they might feel considerable anger or resentment at finding themselves in this new role, suddenly expected to reorientate themselves and their life around an illness. Many struggle with whether or not they can maintain their relationship in the face of the new demand, while others feel neglected and themselves abandoned by their partner, who is receiving a great deal of attention, albeit for a very difficult reason. Probably the most common feeling of all is an immense desire to be able to make things better or to make the pain go away, along with a deep sense of inadequacy and impotence at being unable to achieve this. Sometimes supporters have confessed that they wished their partner could die more quickly so that they personally did not have to keep experiencing such terrible emotional pain.

Of course, these feelings are often mixed with a wonderful sense of new closeness, created by dealing intimately with each other's needs and vulnerability, and there is often a rekindling of great love between partners faced with the possibility of being separated. Many supporters feel very fulfilled in the role, some even feeling that it has brought new purpose and meaning to their lives.

Most people tend to swing between these poles; however personally enriching the positive feelings are, the combination of the emotional intensity, physical and financial demands, added pressures of taking on some of the other's tasks, and getting to and from medical appointments, as well as holding down a job and dealing with the emotional upheaval in the immediate social circle, can be utterly exhausting.

Another problem is that, almost inevitably, both the supporter and the person with cancer try to protect each other from the full impact of what they are feeling, physically and emotionally. This can lead to a protective impasse or double bind, which limits communication and damages relationships. Many supporters have said that their own emotional state tends to mirror that of the person they are caring for, so that they can feel happy and relaxed only when their partner is feeling this way. This leaves them feeling like a cork bobbing about on a sea of emotion, very much at the mercy of what is happening to the other person. Some cope by seeking refuge outside the house – taking trips alone or with friends, or 'escaping' to the cinema or theatre – in order to get a break from the emotional intensity. Many feel that they can never get the pressure of the cancer out of their minds, and while some welcome the lifestyle changes that the cancer can bring with it (especially when the person with cancer makes positive changes through the use of the Bristol Approach), others resent these bitterly.

The other side of the story is that people with cancer often complain that their supporter is inhibiting their emotional expression because they are obviously fed up and no longer able to cope. They also speak about feelings of suffocation from the over-protectiveness of partners, saying that from the moment of diagnosis they have been handled with kid gloves.

From listening to supporters talking in this way, it became clear to us at the Bristol Cancer Help Centre that the combination of stress, exhaustion, emotional conflict and the lack of opportunity to express their feelings was rendering them very vulnerable. It was also apparent that often the relationships between supporters and those they supported were deteriorating because of communication difficulties. This, combined with the social limitations placed on somebody who is increasingly confined to the home base in a care-giving role, puts them at risk of developing stress-related illness themselves, as well as making it likely that their social and professional life will suffer.

Getting Help: The Importance of Counselling

If the provision of support services for people with cancer in the NHS is patchy, to say the least, the provision of support services for supporters is non-existent. There is some minimal recognition by the government of the role of support-givers in the family among the chronically physically or mentally disabled, but almost no recognition of the role families play in looking after somebody who has cancer. This makes it even more vital that people in the support-giving role think very clearly about their own needs and well-being.

If you are a supporter, start by temporarily taking your attention off the loved one. Seek the support of a counsellor, and begin to feel properly the effect that the diagnosis of cancer in one so close has had upon you. For some people this is more easily done without the presence of their partner; indeed, some supporters come to Bristol on their own, and many undertake counselling elsewhere.

The next thing – in exactly the same way as for the person with cancer (whether at the Bristol Cancer Help Centre or not) – is to go through the process of recognizing your own state and needs, with the help as appropriate of doctors, counsellors and healers. If you are able to attend the Centre's five-day course you will also receive bodywork, and will be encouraged to learn the self-help skills of relaxation and meditation so that you can practise these regularly at home in order to protect yourself from the effects of stress. If you are not coming to the Centre, try to get similar help in your home area.

You can use this time to unburden yourself emotionally and to check with a doctor that your physical health is holding up. You might wish to go further, seizing the opportunity that the crisis has given you to think about making lifestyle changes that would be even more protective in the long term. In this way you can engage in a process that mirrors that of the person you are supporting, and become equally excited about the possibilities of making important life-enhancing changes.

Once you have laid these foundations, the most pressing need is to establish regular counselling on a weekly or fortnightly basis. It can also be helpful to have regular healing or massage to deal with the effects of tension and exhaustion.

It is important not to forget the effects on other members of your household. Children, in particular, may be feeling the effects of the stress and distress much more than they say, or even realize themselves. Veronica Mills, who was quoted in Chapter 4, found that she coped with this by asking her own counsellor to do one session a month at the family home with all members of the family present. This gave her children and husband a chance to 'empty out' their feelings on a regular basis. It included once, she told me, her young son's expressing his fury that she was getting a new juicer when he couldn't have a new bike! More seriously, they were enabled to speak freely about their worst fears, talking openly about what it would be like if she died, which gave them all the chance to express their deep love for each other.

It is important that supporters and their partners are given separate, confidential counselling sessions so that they can feel comfortable about expressing their feelings. It is also a good idea to have a session together which focuses on your communication and relationship. This can be particularly important where new problems have arisen since the diagnosis, or if you both feel that there have been long-standing communication or relationship problems that may have contributed to the illness's developing in the first place.

Whether or not you are able to go to the Bristol Cancer Help Centre for this kind of counselling and support, it is important for you to set up your own support system in your home area so that you can access help regularly. A local counsellor can be found through the Centre for Transpersonal Psychology or the British Association for Counselling and Psychotherapy, and a healer through the Healer Referral Service (see Appendix 2).

You may well be inclined to think that you don't need this, or that all the family resources should go towards helping the person with cancer. But it is very important to remember what has been said in Chapter 4 about the way that distress ricochets around the family. Your part in helping to prevent this ricochet effect lies in making sure that you are helped to express your distress and pain outside the family system. By doing this you will be a better supporter for your partner, because you will have cleared your own emotional decks. It is also vital that you yourself are protected through what may be a long and complex process. You may find that you actually grow and benefit from the process, and become closer to the one you love – rather than gradually becoming submerged beneath your feelings, hiding from yourself and your partner, and becoming depressed, embittered and progressively more unavailable, all of which makes it far more likely that you will end up with stress-related illness yourself.

These ideas and suggestions are summarized in the 'Supporter Survival Plan' below.

Supporter Survival Plan

Get Emotional Support
Get yourself a local counsellor. Set up regular visits, even if these are at relatively long intervals, and go for your sessions even if you don't think you need them.

Set yourself up with a personal support team distinct from that of your partner. Meet regularly with your team so that you can talk freely about your needs and what you are going through.

Get joint counselling help if your relationship with the person you are supporting is getting into difficulties.

Take Space and Time for You
Make sure that you don't lose or abandon yourself in the process of looking after the person you are supporting. Create your own private space in the house, and mark out times during the week when you can be on your own – either in or out of the house – pursuing entirely your own interests, or simply resting and relaxing.

Stay Fit
Exercise regularly two or three times a week. Make at least one of these times exercise in the fresh air. If possible, make another a yoga or tai chi class. Perhaps the third could be a swim or some other form of aerobic exercise.

Eat well; if possible, adopt the Bristol Approach to healthy eating, along with your partner.

Take appropriate vitamin and mineral supplements. Contact the Centre's national telephone helpline (see Appendix 2) for their regularly reviewed guidelines.

Develop a Spiritual Practice
If at all possible, commit yourself to learning to meditate. This will give you the inner strength you need to help you to con-

tinue to cope with your situation, as well as benefiting you in other areas of your life.

Remember to pray, too, asking God or the universe to give you the strength you need to meet your challenge.

Keep Communicating

Schedule special times with the person you are supporting so that you can let each other know exactly how you are feeling. This can be very difficult, so it helps if it is done in a structured way: take a specific amount of uninterrupted time each, just to say how you feel. It is immensely tempting to butt in, especially if you feel criticized, or think you have a solution, or simply want to make the other person feel better; but it is far more beneficial – for both of you – if you allow each other the space to talk, cry, shout, or do whatever else you need to do, uninterrupted. It is useful to set a boundary on this exercise by putting a limit on the time for each person to talk.

If, through this process, you identify problems that cannot be sorted out between you, take these to a joint counselling session. Ideally, your joint counsellor should not be the counsellor either of you is seeing individually as this can interfere with your individual counselling and unfairly bias the support given.

Don't forget to keep similar communication lines open with other people who are close to you both, or involved in the supporting role.

Take Regular Breaks

As hard as it may seem, it is important for you to get away regularly so that both of you have a rest from both the intensity of your relationship and the overall situation. If the person you are supporting is very ill, then it may be possible to do this by getting a member of their personal support team to come and stay while you are away. It may be possible for the person who is ill to have breaks away from the home base, too, so that this strategy feels balanced.

Keep Your Own Creative Focus Going

Try not to abandon your own projects or creative ideas. You will be far more helpful and fun to be around if you are being stimulated and enjoying other aspects of your life.

Keep a Journal

Difficult though this period may be, it is a special time of heightened insight and personal growth. Recording your thoughts and feelings is a protective and liberating exercise.

Ask for Help

Do not try to keep everything going on your own. Recognize when you are getting tired, upset or overwhelmed, and ask friends or healthcare professionals for help.

9
When the Going Gets Tough . . .

This chapter offers suggestions and advice for the 'down' times when everything seems to be going badly, or suddenly getting much worse. It emphasizes the importance of continuing to communicate, with yourself and others, and gives guidance on how to do this. It also suggests how you might prepare for, and get yourself through, times of crisis, including how to get support quickly; how to get help at home; and how to cope with pain and insomnia.

Dealing with Renewed Crisis

It is all too easy, at a time of crisis, to forget what help and resources you have at your disposal, either personally, through family and friends, or via professionals. And yet, inevitably, from time to time on your cancer journey you will 'lose the plot', wondering if you have achieved anything at all through your holistic endeavours; and, at such moments, it is more than ever important to get help from your therapists and/or counsellors. If you are taking part in the Bristol Cancer Help Centre's therapy courses, a follow-up visit to the Centre would be appropriate. You can also get help over the phone from the Centre's national telephone helpline.

It is at such 'crisis points' that the work you put in during your initial explorations of the Bristol Approach will pay off immensely. If you have located a good counsellor, healer and energy therapist in your area, they will be there to call upon if things become difficult for you again. This means that you can quickly step up the level of support, knowing not only that these good people are close at hand but also that they already know you well and will be able to go straight to the point.

Troubled times can give fresh impetus to your therapy, taking it to a new, deeper level, which can bring great rewards. The trigger to restart your therapy may be problems in your personal life, new symptoms of the illness or side-effects from treatment, or the news that you have a recurrence. Whether or not it is cancer-related, if you recognize that you have become stressed or distressed then it is time to step up the level of help again.

It is also at difficult times that you will benefit especially from having put time and energy into learning relaxation, meditation and visualization. This remains true even if you are suddenly panicked or thrown into confusion or pain, and feel that these skills have completely deserted you. This is the point at which to loop back round and start the support process all over again – although, in reality, it won't be starting all over again because it will feel like revisiting old friends rather than meeting new people. Once you are back in your support group, or your relaxation or meditation class, or working with your counsellor on the process of visualization, it will all come back to you very quickly; and, again, the opportunity will be there to deepen and intensify your practice.

Keeping in Touch

Communicating with Your Therapist
If you have been through counselling once, and gone quite fully into the Bristol Approach, you might feel that you have 'been

Tuning in

If you find it difficult to 'let go' sufficiently to be able to explore and 'feel' your feelings, it can help if you actively set the stage for it. The way of doing this will vary from person to person, but as time goes on you will discover what works best for you. You could try, for example, running yourself a hot, perfumed bath, lighting a candle and playing some emotionally cathartic music. In these safe but evocative surroundings you can really allow yourself to cry or groan, 'bottoming out' with your pain, distress and anguish.

At first this might seem a scary thing to do: you might feel that if you begin to let go, there will be no end to the release of the feelings stored up inside, and that you will fall into a bottomless pit. However, most people find that after a good ten-minute cry, or a five-minute, full-blast rant, there is very little else to come out. Afterwards, you can enjoy the feeling of 'peace after the storm' when you can 'cuddle' and soothe yourself in a very gentle way, perhaps by curling up under your duvet or by getting a friend to hold or stroke you.

there, done that', and therefore reached a point at which there is nothing more to do. In fact, this is very far from the truth, and it is good to remember Penny Brohn's most pertinent comment that 'healing is a process and not an event'. Much as we would wish it otherwise, life and cancer alike can throw us googlies at any time, knocking us off balance. The most important thing is that you do not deny yourself access to your therapist. Do not fall back into the old habit of thinking that you cannot justify spending the money on yourself in this way, or that you have taken quite enough of their time and attention in the past, or that you had better just buckle down and get on with life.

Communicating with Yourself

Once again, the key issue is about recognizing your state and evaluating your needs (discussed in Chapter 6). Try to do this at any point when your equilibrium is disturbed. Get used to tuning in to how you really feel, taking time to settle down and get in touch with what is going on with your body, your mind and your spirit. You may wish to ask your higher self for insight and guidance: imagine yourself as your own guardian angel, looking at yourself with great love, and seeing from this compassionate perspective more clearly what is needed.

In fact, it is a good idea to get into the habit of tuning into your state regularly (see box on p. 212), either alone, or with a loved one or friend, so that you get better and better at seeing what is going on underneath the coping front that you show the world. This will enable you to adjust your activities and expectations accordingly (if this is necessary), and organize life around your current needs and feelings. Remember that your feelings are always subject to change, and that outer adjustments are not always necessary.

Communicating with Others

When you are under extreme stress it is easy to forget to communicate properly with others about how you are feeling and what you need; yet keeping communication going is vital, even if it is only to tell everybody to leave you alone for a few hours.

If you have constructed a support group of personal friends, this can be a very good time to call an emergency support group meeting in order for them to give you the emotional holding you require to express your feelings. Many people feel the need of the presence of others in order to express their emotions; most of us, initially at least, find it difficult to do on our own in the way described in the box on page 212. At these times you will recognize the value of having built your personal support team prior to getting into difficulties, as it is very hard to make this kind of practical arrangement when you are in trouble.

Of course, the other thing to remember is that if you are going through a difficult time, those close to you are also very likely to feel frightened and upset, and will need support in their own right. The more quickly each of you can take your distress outside of the family or home situation to professional helpers, the quicker the tension levels in the home will start to settle, helping the crisis to pass rather than to escalate. (See Chapter 8 for more on support for carers.)

Bringing Help to You

Sometimes there are practical problems that prevent your being able to get to therapists, groups or classes, and at these times the 'absent healing' services of the National Federation of Spiritual Healers (NFSH) can be invaluable. This organization can be contacted either by phone or in writing. They will ask you for the details of your situation, and then at regular intervals the group of healers who meet to send absent healing will concentrate on sending healing to you. If you have mentioned that those around you are also in trouble, they will send healing to those people as well. Almost always this extraordinary intervention makes a very great difference to your morale, and other help can begin to come in unexpected ways.

It may be that your own healer or therapist is in a position to visit your home; if not, the referral services provided by the NFSH may be able to find a healer who can visit you.

Sometimes a good source of help can be your local church. Even if you are not religious, the local vicar or senior church members are usually very glad to visit the homes of those who are ill or suffering; they are happy just to be there for you, giving comfort, or conducting prayer or services in the house if you would like that. It is also possible to ask friends or your local church to set up a prayer circle for you.

Another very important thing to remember is to pray yourself. Even if you have never prayed in your life before, try asking very specifically for the help you need. Your prayers do not have to be addressed to God; allow yourself to surrender to a force that is greater than you and that can bring you help at your time of need. You may very well be surprised by what can start to come towards you if you let go in this way, and allow yourself to ask for the help you need so badly.

In extremis, the other organization that is absolutely invaluable is the Samaritans, who are there to talk to anyone who is completely at the end of their tether, whatever the problem. Their phone number is prominently displayed in all telephone directories. You can also obtain help from your GP, the practice nurses, the local Macmillan or Marie Curie service, the local hospice or the specialist counsellors on your cancer unit. Don't forget that these services are not set up only for people who are terminally ill or in the midst of a medical emergency; they are available for you whatever difficulties you are experiencing. This is particularly true of modern-day hospices, which usually aim to provide help and support for people with cancer in a whole host of practical and social ways, from the point of diagnosis onwards.

Keeping Control

When the going gets tough the most important thing is to try not to lose yourself or 'give away your power' by 'handing yourself over' to the medical profession. The best way to keep control of your medical situation is by asking for time to think about what you want to do about whatever it is that is being offered to you. This gives you the chance to go through your emotional reaction and gather information, to seek a second opinion medically if necessary, and, most important of all, to work out what it is that is right for you in the situation.

If you feel that not enough is being done, or that your medical team has 'written you off', it is sometimes possible to secure more help by approaching the problem from a different angle. For example, when Penny Brohn's oncology team felt that they could offer no more treatment for her spinal tumour she sought the opinion of an orthopaedic surgeon. When he felt he could offer no help, she sought the opinion of a neurosurgeon. The neurosurgeon leapt into action, performing surgery to decompress the trapped spinal nerves, which were the cause of her increasing difficulty in walking. As a result, Penny had three more years of mobility, and this allowed her to renovate a beautiful mountainside cottage in Crete with her husband David; she created many gorgeous mosaics on the walls and floors, thoroughly enjoying and expressing herself in the process. Without her persistent, lateral approach, she would probably have been bedridden at home or in a hospice receiving palliative care.

As Penny's experiences show, knowing which options can be pursued is part of the battle, and this can be helped considerably if you have a good GP or holistic doctor ally.

Another door that can open wider the harder you push is that giving access to pain management. Usually cancer pain is managed by the GP or palliative care team, but if this is not working it may be time to seek the help of an anaesthetist. Most big cities have pain clinics within their hospitals' departments of anaesthesis, and these can offer very sophisticated pain management which is beyond the scope of most oncology services. For example, if pain has become chronic and unbearable it may be possible for an anaesthetist to perform a permanent pain-block.

Keeping Going

Sometimes it is the nights that are the hardest to bear. You may feel reluctant to disturb your family, and may already have had to decamp into another room overnight so as not to disturb your partner. This can be especially miserable if you are then unable to sleep, either through pain or fear or simply because of relative inactivity or steroid treatment. It is very helpful to get yourself set up with distractions such as a portable television, a laptop computer through which you can access the Internet – or even simply a notebook and pen with which you can begin writing a journal of what you are feeling and thinking, as these very quiet periods are often times of great clarity and poignancy.

Another approach is to try to organize a rota of friends who will come and sit with you through the night. They might well find this a surprisingly rewarding time, allowing them to deepen their relationship with you and catch a glimpse of what it is you are really going through. Here, again, it is a question of being brave enough to ask for what you need.

If you are not in a position to provide yourself with technological distractions or human company, another good plan is to obtain a personal stereo with headphones so that you can use these times to listen to beautiful music or poetry, or even to the whole books that are increasingly available on tape and CD for use by the blind.

If you do become limited in your activity, the great challenge is to keep on living creatively within the new constraints rather than getting stuck in the state of regret for what you have lost. Of course, this can usually happen only after a period of appropriate grieving; but none the less, it is important to try to make the transition so that you can fully express and enjoy yourself within your new limits. This is easier said than done, and it is very difficult not to feel bitter and depressed when things seem to be getting progressively harder. And yet at the Bristol Cancer Help Centre we have all witnessed many people who, given the right level of psychological and spiritual support, have kept on rising to and overcoming the new challenges, and who have continued to find the humour and opportunity in the difficulties while developing ever sweeter, more poignant relationships with themselves and those who care for them.

Suggestions for the 'Down' Days

It is especially important to be able to give to ourselves on the days when we are feeling 'down' or exhausted. Plan a few treats for such times, adding your own favourites to the following suggestions:

- Let go of any plans for the day, telling yourself it really is all right just to rest and nurture yourself.
- Try talking to your body, letting it know that it is strong and can heal and revitalize itself.
- Listen to your favourite music.
- Take a warm bath with aromatherapy oils and candles.
- Buy yourself some flowers.
- Cuddle a soft toy or pillow for comfort.
- Give yourself a treat to eat.
- Burn an uplifting aromatherapy oil like bergamot or clary sage.
- Treat yourself to the type of gentle, loving care you would give if you were looking after a poorly child.
- Go for a short walk and really look at a tree or flower; listen to the birdsong or the wind. If you don't feel well enough to go out, you could sit by a window and do this.
- Tell someone how you are feeling and let him or her help either just by listening, or in some practical way.
- If you feel angry or upset with someone or something, write it out as a letter – which you may or may not wish to send – or do a drawing to express your feelings.
- Imagine that you are being bathed in a gentle healing light of whatever colour feels comfortable to you. Really relax into this – it may lull you into a restful sleep.
- Read some of the inspiring and spiritually uplifting quotes you have collected in your notebook.
- Remember that 'this too will pass' – and tomorrow may find you feeling much brighter.

- You might like to prepare in advance for these 'down' days by creating a 'Rainy Day Box'. A shoebox would do. It might include favourite music and relaxation tapes; a humorous book or video – or anything else which makes you laugh; a food treat; letters or cards from well-wishers which give you pleasure to read; a little book of uplifting quotations. Just include whatever appeals to you and helps you to feel good or gives consolation.

Epilogue:
An Invitation

The almost universal cry from those who have attended a course at the Bristol Cancer Help Centre has been: 'Why, oh why, did I have to get cancer before I could discover this absolutely wonderful process of getting my life and health back on track?' Many have said that everyone should have the opportunity of learning about, and embarking on, the holistic approach to health. And, of course, there is no reason why everyone shouldn't. The Bristol Approach described in this book is as relevant for those wishing to prevent cancer – or simply to enjoy a higher quality of life and health – as it is for those wishing to heal it.

So whether you are reading this book as someone with cancer, as a supporter of someone with cancer, or simply as someone who would like to take steps towards preventing cancer, the crucial step is to commit yourself to embarking upon the holistic approach to health. As is the case with most things in life, the most important – and sometimes the most difficult – step is the first. But, in committing yourself to your life and your health, you will find that the benefits are directly proportionate to your input.

This is perhaps best summed up in Goethe's famous words on the subject of commitment:

Until there is commitment, there is hesitancy.
The chance to draw back, always ineffectiveness.
Concerning all acts of initiative (and creation)
There is one elementary truth, the ignorance of which
Kills countless ideas and splendid plans:
That the moment that one definitely commits oneself,
Then providence moves too.
All sorts of things occur to help one that would never
Otherwise have occurred.
A whole stream of events issues forth from the decision
Raising in one's favour all manner of unforeseen
Incidents and meetings and material assistance,
Which no man could have dreamed would have come his way.
Whatever you can do or dream you can, begin it.
Boldness has genius, power and magic in it.
Begin it now.

We at the Bristol Cancer Help Centre encourage you whole-heartedly to take the crucial steps described in this book to improve your own health and well-being; and we wish you all power, courage, blessings, and our love, as you embark on your own unique healing journey.

References

1   C. B. Pert, M. R. Ruff, R. J. Weber and M. Herkenham, 'Neuropeptides and their receptors: a psychosomatic network', *Journal of Immunology*, 135, 1985, pp. 820–6; Candace Pert, *Molecules of Emotion*, Pocket Books, 1997.
2   H. Goodare, ed., *Fighting Spirit: The Stories of Women in the Bristol Breast Cancer Survey*, Scarlet Press, 1996.
3   L. G. Walker et al., 'Psychological, clinical and pathological effects of relaxation training and guided imagery during primary chemotherapy', *British Journal of Cancer*, 80, 1999, pp. 262–8.
4   A. J. Cunningham et al., 'A prospective, longitudinal study of the relationship of psychological work to duration of survival in patients with metastatic cancer', *Psychooncology*, 9, 2000, pp. 323–39. Also *The Healing Journey: Overcoming the Crisis of Cancer*, Key Porter Books, 2000; *Helping Yourself: A Workbook for People Living with Cancer*, www.healingjourney.toronto.on.ca.
5   J. Griffin and I. Tyrrell, 'The human givens', *The Therapist*, 1998, no. 1. On humour, see N. Cousins, 'Anatomy of an illness (as perceived by the patient)', *New England Journal of Medicine*, 1976, pp. 1458–63; on meaning, see Viktor Frankl, *Man's Search for Meaning*, Pocket Books/Simon & Schuster, 1985; on positive consultations in general practice, see K. and H. B. Thomas, 'General practice consultations: is there any point in being positive?', *British Medical Journal*, 294, 1987, pp. 1200–2;

on the role of emotions, see G. James, L. Yee, G. Harshfield, S. Blank and T. Pickering, 'The influence of happiness, anger and anxiety on the blood pressure of borderline hypertensives', *Psychosomatic Medicine*, 48: 7, 1986, p. 502; on holistic, complementary and creative approaches, see J. Barraclough, ed., *Integrated Cancer Care*, Oxford University Press, 2001; on creativity and writing as therapy, see T. Greenhalgh, 'Writing as therapy', *British Medical Journal*, 319: 31, 1999, pp. 270–1.

6 Lydia Temoschok with H. Dreher, *The Type C Connection: The Behavioral Links to Cancer and Your Health*, Random House, 1992.

7 D. L. Tusek, 'Guided imagery: a significant advance in the care of patients undergoing elective colorectal surgery', *Diseases of the Colon and Rectum*, 40: 2, 1997, pp. 172–8. For guided imagery resources, see the Academy for Guided Imagery, www.interactiveimagery.com; for self-care materials, see www.healthyroads.com; for the Mind–Body Medicine Centre, see www.simontoncenter.com.

8 Leon Chaitow, D. Bradley and C. Gilbert, *Multidisciplinary Approaches to Breathing Pattern Disorders*, Churchill Livingstone, 2001.

9 M. Thomas et al., 'Prevalence of dysfunctional breathing in patients treated for asthma in primary care: a cross-sectional survey', *British Medical Journal*, 322, 2001, pp. 1098–1100.

10 M. Shanks et al., 'Chronic stress in elderly carers of dementia patients and antibody response to influenza vaccination', *Lancet*, 353: 1952, pp. 627–63; J. K. Kiecolt-Glaser, 'Immune responsiveness in caregivers of those with Alzheimer's disease', *Psychosomatic Medicine*, 53, 1991, pp. 345–62; R. Glaser, 'Diminished antibody and immune cell response associated with academic stress', *Psychosomatic Medicine*, 54, 1992, pp. 22–9.

11 Peter Nixon, 'The broken heart: counteraction by

SABRES', *Journal of the Royal Society of Medicine*, 86, 1993, pp. 468–71.

12 E. L. Rossi and D. Nimmons, *The 20 Minute Break*, Los Angeles, Tarcher, 1991.

13 L. G. Walker et al., 'Psychological, clinical and pathological effects of relaxation training and guided imagery during primary chemotherapy', *British Journal of Cancer*, 80, 1999, pp. 262–8.

14 Viktor Frankl, *Man's Search for Meaning*, Pocket Books/ Simon & Schuster, 1985.

15 Ian Gawler, *You Can Conquer Cancer*, Hill of Content, 1984.

16 C. B. Pert, M. R. Ruff, R. J. Weber and M. Herkenham, 'Neuropeptides and their receptors: a psychosomatic network', *Journal of Immunology*, 135, 1985, p. 820–6.

17 On the effects of raised cortisol, see Sephton et al., 'Diurnal cortisol rhythm as a predictor of breast cancer survival', *Journal of the National Cancer Institute*, 92: 12, 2000, pp. 994–1000; D. Spiegel et al., 'Effects of psychosocial treatment in prolonging cancer survival may be mediated by neuroimmune pathways', *Annals of the New York Academy of Science*, 840, pp. 674–83; D. Spiegel, J. Bhloom, H. Kraemer and E. Gottheil, 'Effect of psychosocial treatment on survival of patients with metastatic breast cancer', *Lancet*, 14 Oct. 1989, pp. 888–91.

18 M. Watson et al., 'Influence of psychological response on survival in breast cancer: a population based cohort', *Lancet*, 354, 1999, pp. 1331–6.

19 S. Greer and T. Morris, 'Psychological attributes of women who develop breast cancer: a controlled study', *Journal of Psychosomatic Research*, 19, 1975, p. 147.

20 Laurence LeShan, *Cancer as a Turning Point*, Gateway, 1978.

21 Walker et al., see ref. 13.

22 Spiegel et al., see ref. 17.

23 F. I. Fawzy, et al., 'A structured psychiatric intervention for cancer patients, II: changes over time in immunological measures', *Archives of General Psychiatry*, 47, 1990, pp. 729–35.

24 Naras Bhat, *How to Reverse and Prevent Heart Disease and Cancer*, New Editions Publishing, 1995.

25 Heart Math Publications and Software, http://heartmath.com; Better Physiology Instruments@betterphysiology.com and mindbody@bp.edu.

26 Cunningham et al., 'A prospective longitudinal study of the relationship of psychosocial work to duration of survival in patients with metastatic cancer'.

27 B. Somers and I. Gordon-Brown, *Journey in Depth: A Transpersonal Perspective*, Archive Publishing, 2002.

28 B. Gabriel, E. Bromberg, J. Vandenbovenkamp, P. Walka, A. Kornblith and P. Luzzatto, 'Art therapy with adult bone marrow transplant patients in isolation', *Psycho-oncology*, 10, 2001, pp. 114–23.

29 S. Burns et al., 'A pilot study into the therapeutic effect of music therapy at a cancer help centre', *Alternative Therapies in Health and Medicine*, 7: 1, 2001, pp. 48–56; Leslie Bunt and Sarah Hoskyns, eds, *The Handbook of Music Therapy*, Routledge, 2002, ch. 14.

30 M. Dixon, 'Does healing benefit patients with chronic symptoms? A quasi-randomised trial in general practice', *Journal of the Royal Society of Medicine*, 9: 4, 1988, pp. 183–8.

31 J. Astin et al., 'The efficacy of distant healing: A systematic review of randomised trials', *Annals of Internal Medicine*, 132, 2000, pp. 903–10.

32 Deane Juhan, *Job's Body*, Station Hill, 1994; Lucy Lidell, Sara Thomas et al., *The Book of Massage*, Ebury Press, 1984, rev. edn 2000.

33 Gayle MacDonald, *Medicine Hands*, Findhorn Press, 1999.

34 Patricia Macnamara, *Massage for People with Cancer*, London, Wandsworth Cancer Support Centre, 1994.

35 Patricia Macnamara, see ref. 34.

36 Jennifer Barraclough, *Integrated Cancer Care: Holistic, Complementary and Creative Approaches*, Oxford University Press, 2001.

37 Patricia Macnamara, see ref. 34.

38 Tiffany Field, 'Massage therapy for immune disorders', in Grant Jewell Rich, ed., *Massage Therapy: The Evidence for Practice*, Mosby (Harcourt Publishers), 2002.

39 Silvana Lawvere, 'The effect of massage therapy in ovarian cancer patients', in Rich, ed., *Massage Therapy*.

40 Buford Lively et al., 'Massage therapy for chemotherapy-induced emesis', in Rich, ed., *Massage Therapy*.

41 World Cancer Research Fund (WCRF) in association with American Institute for Cancer Research, *Food, Nutrition and the Prevention of Cancer: A Global Perspective*, 1997. Available from WCRF, 105 Park Street, London, W1Y 3FB.

42 M. Thorogood et al., 'Risk of death from cancer and ischaemic heart disease in meat and non-meat eaters', *British Medical Journal*, 308, 1994, pp. 6945–7012.

43 J. Cummings and S. Bingham, 'Diet and the prevention of cancer: a clinical review', *British Medical Journal*, 317, 1998, pp. 1636–40.

44 J. Plant, *Your Life in Your Hands: Understanding, Preventing and Overcoming Breast Cancer*, Virgin Books, 2002.

45 J. Y. Li et al., 'Nutrition trials in Linxian (multiple vitamin/mineral supplementation, cancer incidence and disease specific mortality among adults with oesophageal dysplasia)', *Journal of the National Cancer Institute*, 85: 18, 1993, pp. 1492–8.

46 N. J. Gonzalez and L. L. Isaacs, 'Evaluation of pancreatic proteolytic enzyme treatment of adenocarcinoma of the

pancreas, with nutrition and detoxification support',
Nutrition and Cancer, 33: 2, 1999, pp. 117–24.

47 J. Barraclough, *Integrated Cancer Care*, p. 158.

48 L. G. Walker et al., 'Relaxation and hypnotherapy: long-
term effects on the survival of patients with lymphoma',
Psycho-oncology, 9, 2000, pp. 355–6.

49 L. B. Seaward, *Managing Stress: Principles and Strategies
for Health and Wellbeing*, Jones & Bartlett, 1994.

50 T. Pinner and C. Pinner, *Into the Silence: A Handbook for
Meditation*, The Healing Sanctuary (Llnaybyther,
Camarthenshire), 1998.

51 J. Macbeth, *Sun over Mountain*, Gateway Books, 1991.

52 Pinner and Pinner, *Into the Silence*; I. Gawler, *You Can
Conquer Cancer*, new edn, Hill of Content, 2001.

53 Deepak Chopra, *Quantum Healing*, Bantam, 1989.

54 K. Luebbert, B. Dahme and M. Hasenbring, 'The
effectiveness of relaxation training in reducing treatment-
related symptoms and improving emotional adjustment in
acute non-surgical cancer treatment: a meta-analytical
review', *Psycho-oncology*, 10, 2001, pp. 490–502; C. X.
Pan, R. S. Morrison, J. Ness, A. Fugh-Berman and R. M.
Leipzig, 'Complementary and alternative medicine in the
management of pain, dyspnea, and nausea and vomiting
near the end of life: a systematic review', *Journal of Pain
and Symptom Management*, 20: 5, 2000, pp. 374–87.

55 R. Sloman, 'Relaxation and the relief of cancer pain',
Nursing Clinics of North America, 30: 4, 1995, pp.
697–709; Luebbert et al., 'The effectiveness of relaxation
training'.

56 Luebbert et al., see ref. 55.

57 T. Burish, M. Carey, M. Krozely and F. Greco,
'Conditioned side effects induced by cancer chemotherapy:
prevention through behavioural treatment', *Journal of
Consulting and Clinical Psychology*, 55: 1, 1987, pp.
42–8; Luebbert et al., see ref. 55.

58 D. Mast, J. Meyers and A. Urbanski, 'Relaxation techniques: a self-learning module for nurses: Unit 1', *Cancer Nursing*, 10: 3, 1987, pp. 141–7.

59 A. Ferrell-Torry and O. Glick, 'The use of therapeutic massage as a nursing intervention to modify anxiety and the perception of cancer pain', *Cancer Nursing*, 16: 2, 1993, pp. 93–101; J. Stringer, 'Massage and aromatherapy on a leukaemia unit', *Complementary Therapies in Nursing and Midwifery*, 6, 2000, pp. 72–6.

60 M. Bredin, 'Mastectomy, body image and therapeutic massage: a qualitative study of women's experience', *Journal of Advanced Nursing*, 29: 5, 1999, pp. 1113–20; Stringer, 'Massage and aromatherapy on a leukaemia unit'.

61 S. Gabriel, *Breathe for Life*, Hardie Grant, 2000.

62 S. C. Paul and G. M. Collins, *Inneractions: Visions to Bring Your Inner and Outer Worlds into Harmony*, HarperSanFrancisco, 1992.

63 Paul and Collins, *Inneractions*.

64 D. Glouberman, *Life Choices and Life Changes: Develop Your Personal Vision with Imagework*, Thorsons, 1995.

Appendix 1
Nutrition and Cancer:
The Bristol Cancer Help Centre Guidelines

Recommended Food and Drink

- Wholefoods, e.g. wholemeal bread, brown flour, brown rice.
- Fresh fruit and vegetables in season, lightly steamed or as salad – try to eat both daily.
- Raw cereals (muesli), nuts, seeds, dried fruits etc. Try to eat some daily.
- Organically grown food, as available and affordable.
- Beans, pulses, lentils, vegetables and cereals. These foods are also a good source of dietary fibre, but bran should be avoided as it is too irritant to the bowel.
- Cold pressed oils for cooking and dressings.
- Freshly made fruit and vegetable juices, using organic fruit and vegetables if possible.
- Lots of filtered or spring water – 2 litres daily is a good goal. Try to drink between meals to avoid filling yourself up with liquid at mealtimes.

In general, go for variety; try to avoid overdependence on one or just a few foods.

Food and Drink to Avoid, in General

- Red meat, i.e. beef, pork, lamb and veal.
- Saturated fat, e.g. milk, cheese, cream and yoghurt (substitute soya products).
- Smoked and salt-cured foods.
- Refined sugar, i.e. any crystal form of sugar (use honey instead).
- Processed and refined foods (they will always contain preservatives and additives, salt and sugar).
- Caffeine in coffee, tea, chocolate and cola drinks.
- Excess alcohol.
- Sweet fizzy drinks.

How you feel about your food and whether you are enjoying it is very important – so there is no need to let your eating become a penance!

Give yourself time to eat slowly, enjoy your meals and relax afterwards if possible.

Where Can I Get More Information on Nutrition?

For more information on nutrition and vitamins, please call the Bristol Cancer Help Centre's national telephone helpline on 0117 980 9505. We will be happy to provide you with our current guidelines regarding vitamin and mineral supplementation. The reason the guidelines are not included in this book is because we review our recommendations regularly as new research emerges. For suggestions on recipes and changing your diet, the Centre has excellent books and videos, written and presented by Jane Sen, our Head Chef and Dietary Adviser:

The Healing Foods Cookbook by Jane Sen
More Healing Foods Cookbook by Jane Sen

Healing foods videos presented by Jane Sen:

> *Delicious and Dairy Free* – how to cook delicious, creamy food without using dairy products;
> *Sweet and Unrefined* – how to cook biscuits, puddings and sweet things without using refined sugar;
> *Juicing and Raw Power* – how to make juices and get more raw food into your diet.

All of these are available from our trading company, CanHelpNow Limited, which you can visit in person, or by mail order via the website on www.canhelpnow.com, or by the 24-hour order line on 0117 980 9522. For enquiries please contact CanHelpNow direct on 0117 980 9504. There is an extensive range of other products and titles available.

Appendix 2
Useful Contacts

The Bristol Cancer Help Centre
Grove House, Cornwallis Grove, Bristol, BS8 4PG

Telephone
Reception: 0117 980 9500
National Telephone Helpline: 0117 980 9505 (our helpline staff are able to offer emotional support and help in finding therapists and support groups in your area)
Bookings: 0117 980 9502

Website
www.bristolcancerhelp.org

Trading Company
The Bristol Cancer Help Centre's trading company, Can Help Now Ltd, stocks a wide range of goods that support a healthy lifestyle. You can obtain these from its shop at the Centre or via mail order. Please ring 0117 980 9500, or visit the website: www.canhelpnow.org

Dr Rosy Daniel
Health Creation: 0117 949 3366

Complementary Cancer Treatments/Information
New Approaches to Cancer: 0800 389 2662
Research Council for Complementary Medicine
(www.rccm.org.uk): 0207 384 1772

Counselling
British Association for Counselling & Psychotherapy (BACP)
(www.counselling.co.uk): 0870 443 5252
Centre for Transpersonal Psychology: 0207 935 7350
National Association of Bereavement Services: 0207 247 1080
UKCP (Counsellors and Psychotherapists): 0207 436 3002
The Cancer Counselling Trust (London-based counsellors):
0207 704 1137
British Association for Behavioural and Cognitive
Psychotherapies: 01254 875277

Healing
The Healer Referral Service: 0845 123 2767
The National Federation of Spiritual Healers: 0845 123 2777

Medical Helplines
CancerBACUP (www.cancerbacup.org.uk): 0808 800 1234
Macmillan Cancerlink (www.cancerlink.org): 0808 808 2020
Breast Cancer Care: 0808 800 6000
NHS Direct: 0845 4647

Nutrition
Institute of Optimum Nutrition: 0208 877 9993
British Association of Nutritional Therapists: 0870 606 1284
The Vegan Society (www.vegansociety.com): 01424 427 393
The Soil Association (where to buy organic food)
(www.soilassociation.org): 0117 929 0661
Argyll Herbs Direct: 01984 624911

Miscellaneous
The Anthroposophical Medical Trust: 01299 861 561
Memorial Sloan-Kettering Cancer Center, New York:
   +1 212 639 4700
American Cancer Society, New York: +1 212 586 8700

Massage
Massage Training Institute (www.massagetraining.co.uk):
   0207 254 7227
British Massage Therapy Council: 0207 323 582

Hypnotherapy
National Register of Hypnotherapists and Psychotherapists:
   01282 716839

Yoga
British Wheel of Yoga: 01529 306 851
The Yoga for Health Foundation: 01767 627 271

Acupuncture
British Council of Acupuncture: 0208 735 0400

Art Therapy
British Association of Art Therapists: 01710 383 3774

Carers
Carers National Association: 0207 490 8818

Homoeopathy
Society of Homoeopaths: 01604 621 400

Music Therapy
Music Space: 0117 976 2634

Reflexology
British Reflexology Association: 01886 821207

Relaxation
Relaxation for Living: 01983 868166

Shiatsu
Shiatsu Society (www.shiatsu.org): 01788 555051

Internet Resources
(Provided by Chrissy Holmes, Bristol Cancer Help Centre Librarian.)
There is a vast amount of information available today on the Internet. How best to evaluate whether a site is of high quality or not can be a problem. By following these simple guidelines, you may save yourself some time.

- Use evaluated gateways like OMNI or Healthfinder.
- Use only approved sites, e.g. those with a Health on the Net (HoN) badge.
- Critically appraise sites yourself – packages like QUICK (Quality Information Checklist) http://www.quick.org.uk are available. It asks:

  (a) Is the information biased?
  (b) Can the information be checked?
  (c) Is it clear who has written the information?
  (d) How current is the web page?

DISCERN – http://www.discern.org.uk – asks 15 key questions to help you see if the information provided is credible and trustworthy. It looks at treatment choices too.

Internet websites are constantly changing and this list is by no means comprehensive.

NB: The contents of the websites listed below *do not* necessarily reflect the opinion of the Bristol Cancer Help Centre; you need to judge for yourself the value of the information given. If in doubt, check with your oncologist.

Cancer Websites

CancerBACUP: Aims to help people live with cancer by providing information and emotional support for patients, and their families and health professionals: http://www.cancerbacup.org.uk

Cancer Directory Online 2002: Created by Macmillan Cancer Relief with input from the Centre for Health Information Quality, it contains information on over 500 cancer resources: http://www.hfht.org/macmillan/index.htm

Cancernet: A service of the US National Cancer Institute, providing access to a database of peer-reviewed summaries on cancer treatment and supportive care: http://www.cancernet.nci.nih.gov

Cancerinfo: Guide to cancer information on the Internet, an excellent place to start searching: http://welcome.to/cancerinfo

Imperial Cancer Research Fund: detailed information on over 30 different types of cancer: http://www.imperialcancer.co.uk

Institute of Cancer Research: in partnership with the Royal Marsden NHS Trust, it is Europe's largest comprehensive cancer centre: http://www.icr.ac.uk

Macmillan Cancer Relief: A UK charity supporting those with cancer and their families: http://www.macmillan.org.uk

National Cancer Institute: USA: http://www.nci.nih.gov

National Electronic Library for Cancer: Provides easy access to best current knowledge about cancer, to improve the care of patients with cancer, and help clinicians and patients make better decisions: http://www.nehl.nhs.uk

WHO International Agency for Research on Cancer: http://www.iarc.fr

Complementary and Alternative Medicine Websites
Acupuncture: http://www.acupuncture.com

British Complementary Medicine Association:
  http://www.bcma.co.uk

Alternative Medicine Foundation: provides information on
  herbs. Links with PubMed for study results:
  http://www.herbmed.org

Consumer Health Information Websites
Acurian: for complete and current disease treatment and
  clinical trials information: http://www.acurian.com

Carers Website: http://www.carers.gov.uk

NHS Direct: http://www.nhsdirect.nhs.uk

Self-help groups: http://www.ukselfhelp.info

Telephone Helplines Association: http://www.helplines.org.uk

Drug Information and Pain Control
Pain control: http://www.painsupport.co.uk

Royal College of Physicians new pain control guidelines:
  http://www.rcplondon.ac.uk/pubs/wp_pc_home.htm

Nutrition
International Bibliography on Dietary Supplements:
  http://www.nal.usda.gov/fnic/IBIDS/index.html

Vegetarian Society: http://www.vegsoc.org

Appendix 3
Further Reading

Many of the books, video tapes and audio tapes listed here are available from the Bristol Cancer Help Centre Shop, on 0117 980 9504, or online (www.bristolcancerhelp.org). ISBN numbers are given at the end of each entry.

Books

Nutrition
Dr Paul Clayton, *Health Defence*, Accelerated Learning Symptoms, Bucks (2001), 0 905 553632

J. Plant, *Your Life in Your Hands: Understanding, Preventing and Overcoming Breast Cancer*, Virgin Books (2002), 0 753 505967

Jane Sen, *Healing Foods Cookbook*, Thorsons (1996), 0 7225 3322 5

Jane Sen, *More Healing Foods*, Thorsons (2001), 0 00711 8341

C. Wheater, *Juicing for Health*, Thorsons (2001), 0 00710 6912

The Mind–Body Approach
W. Bloom, *The Endorphin Effect*, Piatkus (2001), 0 7499 21587

Laurence LeShan, *Cancer as a Turning Point*, Gateway
(1978), 1 85860 046 4

Paul Martin, *The Sickening Mind*, Flamingo (1997),
0 00 655022 3

Caroline Myss, *Anatomy of the Spirit*, Bantam (1996),
0 553 50527 0

Candace Pert, *Molecules of Emotion*, Pocket Books (1997),
0 671 03397 2

Ian Gawler, *You Can Conquer Cancer*, Hill of Content
(2001), 0 85572 141 3

E. Lewis, R. O. Brier and J, Barraclough (eds), *The Psycho-immunology of Cancer*, 2nd edn, Oxford University Press
(2002), 0 192 630 601

Counselling
B. Somers and I. Gordon-Brown, *Journey in Depth: A
Transpersonal Perspective*, Archive (2002) 0 9542 7120 3

Symptom Management
J. Barraclough, *Integrated Cancer Care: Holistic,
Complementary and Creative Approaches*, Oxford
University Press (2001), 0 19 2630954

Meditation
Ian Gawler, *Peace of Mind*, Prism Press (1989),
1 85327 027 X

Full Kabat-Zinn, *Catastrophic Living: How to Cope with
Stress, Pain and Illness Using Mindfullness Meditation*,
Piatkus (1990), 0 7499 15854

Laurence LeShan, *How to Meditate*, Thorsons (1995),
1 85538 277 6

Healing
Larry Dossey, *Healing Words*, HarperCollins (1994),
0 06 250252 2

Deepak Chopra, *Quantum Healing*, Bantam (1989),
  0 553 173332 4

Massage
Patricia Macnamarra, *Massage for People with Cancer*, Cancer
  Resource Centre, Wandsworth (1994), 0 95232243 9

Pain
Neville Shone, *Coping Successfully with Pain*, Sheldon Press
  (1992), 0 85969 750 9

Death and Dying
Elisabeth Kübler-Ross, *Wheel of Life*, Bantam (1998),
  0 553 50544 0
Stephen Levine, *Healing into Life and Death*, Gateway
  (1987), 0 946551 48 0
Stephen Levine, *Meetings at the Edge*, Gateway (1984),
  0 946551 88 X
Ed Nicholls, Gill Elliot and Joseph Elliott, *New Natural
  Death Handbook*, Rider Books (1997), 0 7126 7111 0
Sogyal Rinpoche, *Tibetan Book of Living and Dying*, Rider
  Books (1992), 0 7126 7139 0

Alternative Cancer Medicines
W. Diamond, John Cowden, W. Lee and Burton Goldberg,
  Definitive Guide to Cancer, Future Medicine Publishing
  Inc., 88729901 7

Visualization
Jeanne Auchterberg, *Imagery in Healing*, Shamballa (1985),
  0 394 73031 3
Shakti Gawain, *Creative Vizualization*, Bantam (1978),
  0 553 27044 3
Ian Gawler, *Creative Power of Imagery*, Hill of Content
  (1997), 0 85572 281 9

J. Macbeth, *Sun over Mountain*, Gateway (1991),
   0 7171 33885
Carl Simonton, *Getting Well Again*, Bantam (1988),
   0 553 28033 3

Audio Cassettes and CDs

Meditation
Jenni Adams, *Inner Silence*
Jenni Adams, *Meditation Made Easy*

Relaxation
Jenni Adams, *Relax and Sleep Well*
Christopher Greatorex, *Relaxation and Visualisation First
   Steps* (BCHC tape)
Barbara Siddall, *Moving Stillness*

Yoga
Barbara Siddall, *Altered States 1*
Tessa Morgan, *Yoga at Home*

*(All Jenni Adams tapes from 'Mind Your Body Cassettes' can
be bought from the BCHC shop.)*

Index